Home Birth

A PRACTITIONER'S GUIDE TO BIRTH OUTSIDE THE HOSPITAL

Contributors

George J. Annas   Judith Dickson Luce

Jenifer M. Fleming   Elizabeth Noble

Home Birth

A PRACTITIONER'S GUIDE TO BIRTH OUTSIDE THE HOSPITAL

Stanley E. Sagov, M.D.
Department of Family and Community Medicine
University of Massachusetts

Richard I. Feinbloom, M.D.
Department of Family Medicine
State University of New York at Stony Brook

Peggy Spindel, R.N.
Chairperson, Massachusetts Midwives' Alliance
Newton, Massachusetts

with

Archie Brodsky
Boston, Massachusetts

WQ
415
.S129
1984

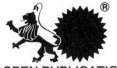

1 0 8 6 7

AN ASPEN PUBLICATION®
Aspen Systems Corporation
Rockville, Maryland
Royal Tunbridge Wells
1984

Library of Congress Cataloging in Publication Data

Sagov, Stanley E.
Home birth.

"An Aspen publication."

Includes index and bibliographies.
1. Childbirth at home. I. Feinbloom, Richard I. II. Spindel,
Peggy. III. Title. [DNLM: 1. Delivery—Methods.
WQ 415 S129h]
RG652.S24   1984   618.4   83-15671
ISBN: 0-89443-947-2

Publisher: John Marozsan
Editorial Director: Darlene Como
Executive Managing Editor: Margot Raphael
Editorial Services: Martha Sasser
Printing and Manufacturing: Debbie Collins

Library of Congress Catalog Card Number: 83-15671
ISBN: 0-89443-947-2

Printed in the United States of America

1   2   3   4   5

Fear is implanted in us as a preservative from evil; but its duty, like that of other passions, is not to overbear reason, but to assist it. It should not be suffered to tyrannize in the imagination, to raise phantoms of horror, or to beset life with supernumerary distresses.

—Samuel Johnson

Table of Contents

Forewords

Home Birth: A Practitioner's Guide to Birth Outside the Hospital is obviously the fruit of long experience in, and hard thinking about, home births. It is a comprehensive introduction to the subject for couples desiring a home birth and for physicians or midwives who wish to start attending home births, and at the same time it can add to the knowledge of the most experienced practitioners.

The authors are fair and charitable in their treatment of physicians trying to stamp out home births. They have written a book for our times. Some things we hope will change. For example, their list of contraindications of home birth is extremely extensive, and some are merely statistical, such as primiparous women over age 35. This is appropriate, as the authors state, for the present day when home birth attendants may be charged with malpractice or even murder for incidents that in a hospital would attract no attention. Perhaps some day conditions with some risk that can be handled as well at home as in a hospital, such as breeches suitable for vaginal delivery, will be explained to the parents and they will pick the place of birth.

The safety of home births is very well covered. The ideal relationships between midwives and physicians and between home birth attendants and consultants are laid out in a most understanding manner. Prenatal care and care of mother and baby during and after birth are succinctly and thoroughly explained.

I hope this book will be widely read. This will benefit the authors as they deserve, home birth practitioners much more, and mothers, babies, and families most of all.

Gregory J. White, M.D.
American College of Home Obstetrics

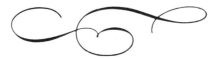

The intensity of feeling that surrounds the issue of birth outside of the hospital is based only partly on reason, and much more on fear. At the turn of the century most deliveries took place at home. Birth attendants were "granny midwives" with no formal training. Nonetheless, many authorities believed that the midwives' results were superior to those of the poorly trained physicians of that era.[1] In the years since, a revolution has occurred. All but a small percentage of deliveries in the United States occur in hospitals, and midwives deliver only 3 percent or so. This change in place of birth and of birth attendant has been associated with a remarkable reduction in maternal and perinatal mortality, but association does not prove causation. The extent to which improvements in maternal and fetal welfare result from a general improvement in standard of living for all, the training of birth attendants, and the provision of prenatal care independent of the change to hospital birth has never been addressed. Out-of-hospital birth is common in several European countries and with good results.[2] Even in our system, many deliveries occur in less well-equipped hospitals and are attended by physicians with considerably less than specialty training in obstetrics and gynecology. There is a great contrast between the kind of technically high quality care that can be provided in the best hospital setting and that which can be provided in the home, but how much contrast is there, really, between a small hospital's care and the well-trained and equipped home delivery team? If the mother can be transported to a hospital within 10 minutes where a team awaits capable of performing an emergency Cesarean section, the outcome of an emergency at home may be better than if the mother were laboring in a small hospital where it would take half an hour to assemble the Cesarean section team. In addition, there is evidence that at the extreme, the cold, overly professional atmosphere of the worst hospital settings may increase obstetric casualties.[3]

On the other hand, physicians and nurses who deliver babies in hospitals know that in obstetrics, "rare" events with adverse outcomes are not that rare. The 25 percent of pregnancies that are recognized in advance as "high-risk" do account for half of the perinatal casualties, but the 75 percent of pregnancies that make up the "low-risk" majority still produce 50 percent of the problems.[4] Most of these problems occur suddenly, and while they can be managed initially out of the hospital part of the time, anyone with experience in obstetrics can remember many almost-tragedies that did not happen because the right people and equipment were available when every second counted.

In addition, there are the medical-legal concerns. Law suits claiming $20,000,000 for the care of a child with cerebral palsy from presumed birth injury are not unheard of these days. All of these considerations lead physicians and hospital nurses to fear innovations in childbirth. There are enough tragedies that occur, even under the very best of circumstances, that seem beyond our ability to prevent with all the skills and instruments at our disposal. To risk increasing what cannot be controlled, knowing we will be held responsible, is terrifying.

As a nation, we have accepted one solution to providing high quality obstetrical care: trained physician specialists delivering in hospitals. A large segment of the public is dissatisfied with this solution as presently practiced. They decry the overly interventive approach to childbirth. They complain about hospital policies that interfere seemingly without benefit. They hear of too many Cesareans and operative deliveries. Most of all, they fear the loss of autonomy that goes with becoming a "patient" in a hospital. They do not want to relinquish control over this exciting part of their lives.

This reviewer presents his own bias, that the best solution is to work to change the hospital delivery suite to make it more like the home. The delivery suite could be a collection of individual birthing rooms that belong for a time to the laboring woman and her family, where they can come to have a baby with good help and safe surroundings, but without relinquishing control. The birthing room would be an extension of the home, where we physicians, midwives, and nurses would come to help with the process, but not to control it. All of the technical support of the hospital would be there, just on the other side of the wall for "emergency use only," but otherwise unseen.

It is harder to change an existing setting than to create a new one. Couples having babies right now want a better birth experience; they have no time to change the system, except by voting to stay out of it. Hence, the growing home birth movement and the rapid rate of establishment of out-of-hospital birth centers.

It is essential that those who want a home birth or who plan to attend births in the home have a guide to help them prepare. For them this book will serve an important purpose. It is written by a group who together have attended many home births and who have thought and planned at length about all of the steps necessary for a safe and rewarding birth experience. Some chapters represent the very distinct opinions of their authors. As the authors have stated, this book is not meant as a complete,

xiv HOME BIRTH: A PRACTITIONER'S GUIDE

impartial review of the literature. It derives from the experiences of the authors and reflects their enthusiasm for the cause. It is not intended to serve in place of a textbook of obstetrics or of thorough professional training. Some might take issue with some of the observations, as, for example, that anxiety can cause labor to stop even when the cervix is widely dilated. However, those who are seriously interested will find here a wealth of helpful information.

Phillip G. Stubblefield, M.D.
Associate Professor of Obstetrics and Gynecology
Harvard Medical School

NOTES

1. Alfred Yankauer, "The Valley of the Shadow of Birth," *American Journal of Public Health* 73 (1983): 635–637.

2. G. David Adamson and Douglas J. Gare, "Home or Hospital Births?" *Journal of the American Medical Association* 243 (1980): 1732–1736.

3. Roberto Sosa et al., "The Effect of a Supportive Companion on Perinatal Problems: Length of Labor and Mother-Infant Interaction," *New England Journal of Medicine* 303 (1980): 597–613.

4. Robert W. Wilson and B.S. Schifrin, "Is Any Pregnancy Low Risk?" *Obstetrics and Gynecology* 55 (1980): 653–656.

Preface

As women's health activists and educators for over a decade, we have been strong advocates of midwives, home birth, and freestanding birth centers, all of which emphasize the essentially healthy, nonmedical nature of childbirth. Several of us in the Boston Women's Health Book Collective have had home births and know firsthand the joys and comforts of having our babies in a warm, familiar setting surrounded by loved ones and skilled, sensitive birth attendants. We also know that all labors that begin at home may not end there and that certain complications may require transfer to a hospital setting to ensure a safe birth for mother and/or baby. However, we believe that the great majority of women who have had normal pregnancies and who would prefer to give birth at home can do so safely without requiring the obstetrical technology available in the hospital setting. Unfortunately, this option is now possible for relatively few women, a situation we hope this book will change by giving medical students, physicians, and midwives a more positive and balanced perspective on home birth in particular and on normal birth in general.

To raise the subject of home birth often evokes horrified cries of "How could you take such a chance with your baby? What if something should go wrong?" Parents choosing home birth are often labeled selfish and irresponsible, the implication being that they are seeking a nice "cozy" experience for themselves at the expense of their baby-to-be. To the contrary, these parents are *extremely* concerned with their baby's safety and well-being. They have usually studied carefully the dangers of hospital birth and have decided that home birth, despite its own set of risks, is the safer choice.

Some would argue that hospitals are changing, that the new "homelike" birthing rooms are humanizing the hospital birth experience. Unfortunately such cosmetic changes mean little in the face of medical training that continues to perpetuate a highly medicalized view of childbirth. Women still commonly endure so much inappropriate treatment in hospitals: restrictions about eating and drinking, routine IVs, opposition to adopting certain labor positions such as squatting or hands and knees, artificial rupturing of membranes, routine fetal monitoring, overuse of artificial augmentation of labor and/or anesthesia, unnecessary use of episiotomy and forceps, and so forth. More important, and even worse than any particular intervention, is the way in which the presence of all this obstetrical technology more often than not erodes a woman's confidence in her own ability to give birth without intervention.

Many hospitals exclude nurse-midwives and family practice physicians, most of whom have a less medicalized approach to birth than obstetricians. Even when nurse-midwives can practice in a hospital, they and their clients often endure inappropriate interference from obstetricians. Midwives in hospitals *do* make a difference, but their numbers are still so small (about 2,000 nurse-midwives nationwide) and their skills so devalued by most obstetricians that most women will never have access in the hospital setting to all that midwifery can offer.

Whether or not current efforts to reform hospitals are ultimately successful, some women and their families will always prefer home birth to hospital birth. We look forward to a time when every community will have the practitioners and resources to be able to offer this option to all families who want it and when women, as midwives, will regain their role as primary attendants for women giving birth, regardless of the setting.

We hope that this well-researched, comprehensive book moves us closer to that time and that it enables useful dialogues to occur among women, their families, and practitioners. Moving beyond the strong emotions surrounding discussions about home birth, the writers of this book sanely examine the most important issues—the woman as the center of her own birth experience, the family's capacity to make responsible choices, communication between family and practitioners, the relationship between doctors and midwives, and the relative safety of home and hospital birth. We are immensely grateful to the authors, midwives and doctors alike, for giving us the benefit of their experience in working together, and we know that their efforts help all of us as we work to make childbirth more satisfying, safe, and humane.

Judy Norsigian and Jane Pincus for the
Boston Women's Health Book Collective

Acknowledgments

The birth of this book has been made possible by many people working together, whether or not their names and their words appear in these pages. The Boston Women's Health Book Collective has supported us in building a physician-midwife practice that in turn could support women in making their childbearing experiences their own. We thank those who have been a part of that service and helped make it work, especially Eric Henley, M.D., Susan Robbins, Laurie Howell, Kathryn Porterfield, R.N., F.N.P., the staff of Family Practice Group, and the medical students whose enthusiastic assistance has carried with it a promise of continuity. From the beginning Lenora Smith has held things together in more ways than we can enumerate. Judith Dickson Luce's contribution to the practice and to the book has extended far beyond the chapter she coauthored.

We are deeply indebted to those who instructed us in low-intervention, family-centered maternity care, including Andrew Elia, M.D., the late John Franklin, M.D., Christina Kielt, C.N.M., Ruth Lubic, Ed.D., C.N.M., Robbie Pfeufer, Pam Putney, C.N.M., Joan Richards, C.N.M., Leo Sorger, M.D., Gregory White, M.D., and Ruth Wilf, C.N.M. No less important is what we have learned from one another in attending births together. Harold Bursztajn, M.D., and Robert Hamm, Ph.D., developed an approach to clinical decision making under conditions of uncertainty, which was then elaborated in a book that two of us wrote with them; it has been a guiding philosophy of our work. David Dowis, M.D., and Janet Dowis, M.D., gave us the benefit of their experience so as to make our data pool larger and more representative. G. J. Kloosterman, M.D., provided an inspiring example through both his published and unpublished work. Fran Ventre, C.N.M., Joan Richards, C.N.M., and Benjamin Chaska, M.D., wrote chapters for this book that, in the end, we did not have space to include. (Interviews with three families about their births suffered the same fate.) Mary Lee Ingbar, Ph.D., M.P.H., explored the economics of our practice in a project supported by the National Fund for Medical Education through a grant sponsored by the American Hospital Supply Corporation. Gail Page and Penny Stratton contributed essential research and logistical support. As if it were not enough to have typed the manuscript, Frances Judkins and her husband Chet added three uncomplicated and joyous home births to our series. Darlene Como, our editor, exercised the skills of a dedicated midwife in guiding the book through a long and difficult gestation. The book is stronger for the critical readings given it by Betty Clarke, Janet Leigh, R.N., Phillip Stubblefield, M.D., and Gregory White, M.D.

We thank those obstetricians and neonatologists who, in spite of differences of opinion, have provided consultation and backup for us and for the families we have worked with; we thank as well those who have joined us in a constructive dialogue by comparing their methods and outcomes with ours. Their commitment to a free exchange and testing of ideas has been heartening. Local groups such as Birth Day, Maternal and Child Health Center, and Homebirth, Inc., have formed a vital support system and information network. Special thanks to the many parents, birth attendants, childbirth educators, and others active in the out-of-hospital birth movement—both the innovators of the current revolution in maternity care and the traditionalists who have been doing it all along. Just knowing that these people and organizations are out there has made us feel part of a community. And to our families, in return for their personal and moral support in this unorthodox endeavor, we hope we can give back something of what we have learned from other families, those who have invited us into their homes to witness their births.

Introduction

This book has been written to conciliate, to reassure, and to establish a substantive basis for discussion of a subject on which more heat than light has been shed. Its purpose is not to proselytize for the home as the preferred site for childbirth but to advocate for the availability of home birth as a reasonable option for properly screened and prepared women attended by qualified practitioners with hospital backup. The authors' clinical experience in a physician-midwife practice in the Boston area, together with the data reviewed in Chapter 2, indicates that home birth is a safe alternative under these conditions—a position endorsed by the International Childbirth Education Association (ICEA)[1] and the American College of Nurse-Midwives (ACNM).[2]

This text, which codifies the experience and methods of a successful home birth service, is addressed to practicing professionals who desire to attend out-of-hospital births or to make informed choices concerning what (if any) part to play in a support system for out-of-hospital birth. The term *professionals* here is broadly construed so as to include physicians and nurses (in obstetrics, family medicine, pediatrics, and other specialities), lay midwives and nurse-midwives, educators and students (in medicine, midwifery, and nursing), childbirth educators, members of the legal professions, and health care policy makers and administrators. This broad potential readership testifies to the cooperative character of home birth, a holistic endeavor that brings into play clinical, logistical, ethical, economic, political, and legal considerations.

In this effort the role of the midwives and physicians who attend births in the home and other out-of-hospital settings is central—less central only than that of the women giving birth and their families. To these practitioners we offer the encouragement of a positive example and propose a set of standards for responsible practice. We aim thereby to encourage more nurse-midwives to work in the home and in alternative birth centers, to legitimize the work of lay midwives, and to gain greater acceptance for home birth as an area of practice for physicians and as a subject of academic scrutiny.

In so doing we must note, with wonder and regret, the fierce controversy that has surrounded this issue—a controversy unlike any other in medicine in its intensity. The advantages of home versus hospital care are being reevaluated in other areas, such as renal dialysis, the treatment of heart attack victims, and the care of the dying patient. Nowhere, however, is there the kind of shrill adversarial exchange found in the home birth debate, in which each side, in effect, accuses the other of killing and maiming mothers and infants, in the one case by neglect and unnecessary risk and in the other by assaultive intervention.

Particularly regrettable, in light of the tradition of scientific and scholarly integrity to which the medical profession subscribes, has been the dismissal of home birth as a legitimate option in the absence of data showing site to be a significant determinant of outcomes of low-risk labors. It is inconceivable that, given the same lack of supporting evidence, medical educators and consultants would take such a moralistic, prohibitive stance toward, for example, coronary bypass grafts or the treatment of diabetes with oral agents. We believe we can best contribute to setting a different tone for the discussion by attempting to delineate what is known about home birth and what is not yet known, what consensus has been reached and what the ranges of disagreement are. We invite other home birth attendants as well as those who oppose home birth to contribute to this dialogue.

* * * * *

Although clinical issues specific to the home site are treated prominently in this text, the underlying attitude toward birth and the approach to labor and delivery are by no means site dependent. In the first place, the same noninterventive philosophy and similar criteria for transfer to hospital are characteristically applied in freestanding birth centers. In the words of Lubic and Ernst, "A childbearing center is an adaptation of the home, rather than a modification of the hospital."[3] Thus, the clinical protocols set forth here can be followed in other out-of-hospital sites as well as in the home.

Furthermore, they can and should be followed within as well as outside the hospital. Although transport during labor is not an issue in planned hospital deliveries (except in occasional transfers to better staffed and equipped facilities), the question of when to intervene in the natural course of labor is still one for which delicately trained clinical judgment is required. The decision whether to continue a trial of labor in a birthing room or to perform a cesarean section, while influenced by the proximity of the operating room, requires consideration of the full range of objective and subjective factors discussed in the context of home birth in Chapter 11.

Reliance on watchful expectancy based on clinical experience rather than routine intervention based on statistical norms implies an attitude that honors the overwhelming likelihood of a normal outcome even as it acknowledges the everpresent possibility of abnormality. In low-risk obstetrics the attendant is a witness and an ally in a natural process that is almost sure to go well irrespective of what the attendant does or does not do. The attendant's role is not, however, adequately defined in negative terms alone. That is, it is not simply a matter of realizing that birth is not a medical emergency and of refraining from unnecessary interventions such as routine anesthesia or episiotomy. The attendant also has the vital positive role—over the prenatal course as well as during and after labor— of reinforcing people's awareness of their health and strength, modeling a hopeful but realistic attitude, guiding the progress of difficult labors, and giving reassurance that apparent abnormalities often resolve themselves in time. While allowing for organic factors that may lead to a bad outcome for the most well-prepared woman (or a good outcome for the least well-prepared), the attendant is also aware that the outcome of labor can be a self-fulfilling prophecy on the part of the woman, her family, or the attendant.

The birth attendant works to enhance the prospective parents' sense of ownership of the process of family formation while taking all reasonable measures to anticipate clinical complications. Part of the responsibility and the pleasure of attending births is to get to know families as well as possible prenatally so as to interpret more sensitively the woman's responses during labor and to assess the significance of deviations from normal labor patterns. This kind of client-attendant relationship makes childbirth not only a time of great moment for the family but also a mutually educative experience. The family learns how to handle every aspect of the birth process, from prenatal nutrition and exercise to preparing the birth room to breast-feeding and early child care. The attendant learns how different individuals and families cope with stress and react to joy. Both learn something new about the physical and emotional capacities of human beings.

This approach to childbirth demands time, effort, and patience from the attendant. For reasons stemming from economic factors and traditions of professional training, it has to date been practiced more regularly in home births than in hospital births and more regularly by midwives and some family physicians than by obstetricians. However, it need not be limited to any particular site or type of practitioner. The attitudes and practices identified with home birth have had and will continue to have a beneficial influence on hospital obstetrics. Hospital practitioners who are dissatisfied with mainstream obstetrics, but who would not consider attending births outside the hospital, may wish to adapt the principles and protocols in this text to the hospital setting through the use of physician-midwife teams.

* * * * * *

The chapters that follow are divided into two sections, which are most usefully read conjointly but may be consulted separately by readers who seek only, on the one hand, an overview of the controversy surrounding home birth, or, on the other, a procedural manual. In Part I, Home Birth in Context, the cultural, philosophical, scientific, legal, economic, political, and logistical implications of home birth are examined. Highlighted in this section are discussions of the safety of home birth and of relationships between midwives and physicians. In Part II, Home Birth in Practice, instruction in safe, medically supervised, family-centered home delivery with hospital backup is provided. Among the skills detailed are screening for eligibility; dynamic assessment of risk; management of normal pregnancy, labor, delivery, and postpartum care; recognition and management of deviations from the norm; indications for transfer to hospital; relationships with consultants; and attentiveness to the needs of the family at all stages of the process.

Although this book is intended as a primary text for home birth attendants and for that purpose contains extensive discussions of prenatal care and of normal labor and delivery, it also assumes prior familiarity with basic texts in obstetrics and midwifery, such as those listed in Appendix C. The reader is assumed to have such texts available and to have had supervised experience in attending normal labors. In this text there is a selective emphasis on clinical issues specifically relevant to the out-of-hospital site, such as prospective evaluation of complications, appropriate responses to unanticipated developments in the home, and effects of time and distance on clinical decisions. For example, in the case of a retained placenta, a hospital practitioner with a noninterventive philosophy may be able to respond more flexibly (i.e., wait longer to remove the placenta) than an attendant in the home who does not have the same resources at hand for instant mid-course corrections.

Finally, this collaboration reflects the creative tension that has helped make the authors' practice work in its own unusual and very gratifying way. There are many questions that physicians and midwives tend to answer differently. To harmonize these differences of opinion and at the same time acknowledge them, we have opted for neither a fully homogenized coauthored text nor chapters credited entirely to individual authors.

Instead, by identifying the "principal authors" of each chapter, we have tried to be faithful to the divergent points of view that make up our practice while making clear that all of us have had a hand in every chapter. As in the births we have attended, the responsibility is shared.

NOTES

1. International Childbirth Education Association, "Position Paper on Planning Comprehensive Maternal and Newborn Services for the Childbearing Year." Seattle, 1979.

2. American College of Nurse-Midwives, "Statement on Practice Settings." Washington, D.C., 1980.

3. Ruth Watson Lubic and Eunice K. M. Ernst, "The Childbearing Center: An Alternative to Conventional Care," *Nursing Outlook* 26 (1978): 754–760.

Part I

Home Birth in Context

Chapter 1

Why Home Birth?

Principal Authors: Judith Dickson Luce, Stanley E. Sagov, M.D., and
Archie Brodsky

The reasons for the revival of home birth in America since the 1970s are well known. Nonetheless, it is worth reviewing them briefly in response to the claim that the establishment of out-of-hospital birth centers and the increasing availability of family-centered birth in hospital "birthing rooms" have made home birth unnecessary. Why have a well-informed, articulate minority of American women and their families returned to the traditional site of birth a generation after the historic shift to hospital birth? What reasons for choosing home birth are valid today? What do families as well as midwives and physicians have to gain from participating in home birth or supporting its availability as an option? Are there possible benefits for the medical profession and for society as well?

ORIGINS OF THE RETURN TO HOME BIRTH

Resurgence of interest in home birth grew out of the confluence of several major social forces—feminism, the prepared childbirth movement, the reassertion of family values, the holistic health movement, and the health consumer movement—all of which focused attention on personal awareness, self-care, and informed choice. Foremost among these in many parts of the country was the women's movement. With the publication of *Our Bodies, Ourselves*[1] in 1971, women individually and collectively sought to reclaim responsibility for their physical well-being from the predominantly male medical profession. Through childbirth education classes and the rediscovery of natural childbirth and breast-feeding, women began to reassert control over an experience that is uniquely theirs.

All of the essential medical detail in this book (much of it pertaining to the recognition and management of complications that occur very infrequently) should not obscure the fact that what shapes the birth experi-

3

ence—what gives it meaning and almost always brings it to a successful conclusion—is the strength that resides in a woman's body and in her self-awareness. Those who attend women in childbirth—regardless of site—should see their medical knowledge as augmenting that strength when needed, rather than as supplanting it or serving some other professional or institutional agenda. We hope that attendants who make use of this book, however medically vigilant they must be, will begin with a profound reverence for the birth process and recognition of the need for caring, watchful patience as a woman in labor finds her own pace, mood, and method. One factor motivating the choice of home birth has been the prevalence of this noninterventive spirit among birth attendants who work in the home.

Women lost control of birth when physicians, who were at that time almost exclusively male, took the place of midwives and female family members or neighbors by the side of the woman in labor. Fittingly, the movement to regain this control on the part of birthing women has stressed the importance of the role of women as primary attendants. Women traditionally have attended other women in childbirth, encircling them, supporting them, empowering them with the strength that came from their own experiences of giving birth. As women have watched other women give birth, they have transmitted the knowledge of birth from generation to generation. Although the continuity of this tradition has been broken in modern Western civilization, it is being restored through the experience and dedication of women who are helping other women understand the workings of their bodies and are thereby also helping women and their male partners become families. Even so, it is not the midwife, but the birthing woman herself, who stands at the center of feminist consciousness concerning birth. It is the woman who gives birth; the midwife or physician simply attends.

The medical model of birth has been challenged not only by women but also by their male partners. Prospective fathers and other close relatives have a stake in the creation of a new family member, and their presence and participation set a tone for the life of the newborn and the future existence of the family as a whole. If the active participation of women in birth is a revival of tradition, that of men is a step into an unknown realm (although there are historical precedents for male involvement in childbirth). Once barred even from observing their children's births, men now share the effort, the responsibility, the emotional stresses and strains, and the revelations (about women and about their own births). Yet as long as hospital regulations reflected outdated cultural patterns by restricting the father's presence in the delivery room, men could give their partners labor support only at home.

NATURE VERSUS TECHNOLOGY IN CHILDBIRTH

The choice of prepared, unmedicated childbirth was one expression of a growing distrust of medical technology in favor of "natural" means to good health, such as diet and exercise. Suzanne Arms in *Immaculate Deception*[2] and Doris Haire in *The Cultural Warping of Childbirth*[3] argued persuasively that unnecessary medical interventions not only disrupt the natural processes (both physiological and psychological) of birth but also can do iatrogenic damage. For example, different forms of anesthesia in varying degrees interfere with the mother's ability to participate actively in her care and consciously be with her partner and family during the birth. She becomes incapable of controlled expulsion in the second stage or of bonding with the newborn. Because the mother cannot actively give birth under anesthesia, the baby may be more likely to be subjected to other potentially harmful interventions. Under some conditions the depressive effect of anesthesia has been observed to leave the baby less sentient, less aware of the environment, and less responsive than a baby born without maternal anesthesia. These effects are the subject of continuing research and may be reduced by the development of new anesthetics. Nonetheless, although there are times when the benefits of anesthesia exceed its costs, its use in childbirth is difficult to justify in the absence of abnormal levels of pain related to a pathological condition.

Any intervention has its price. The uncritical application of technology is unsound because to tamper with any part of the ecosystem is to risk unanticipated and perhaps unknowable effects on other parts of the system—effects that should be risked only for clear benefits, such as saving life or alleviating intense pain. On the other hand, nature is not all bountiful. To leave birth entirely to nature (e.g., by having inadequately attended home births without provision for hospital backup) is to accept rates of preventable death and injury that are unacceptable in Western cultures.

The question of how we accommodate to nature, with and without technology, is more complex than some of the argument on the subject would suggest. The technological, medicalized approach to childbirth, which disregards many of the values of concern to alternative birth advocates, is not itself value free. Depending on how one looks at it, it may be seen to value outcome to the exclusion of process (save the baby at all costs) or else to value a certain kind of process even above outcome (use capital-intensive methods even if these are not the best way to save the baby). At the other extreme, to deny the usefulness of medical technology is to disavow those values that have made human beings unwilling to accept the random, impersonal outcomes of nature—i.e., empathy, morality, kinship ties, and an instinct for survival that motivates us to plan, to improve, to invent, to provide for the future, and to assess causal relationships as well as uncertainties. It is only human to acknowledge that some natural events do not meet human needs. Human beings and their creations are part of nature, and it is part of human nature to conceive technological means for survival as well as to perceive potential dangers to survival inherent in those means.

What is needed is not an allegiance to or rejection of means in themselves but a critical assessment, at any given decision point, of what means best serve human values. Although the "back to nature" theme of the alternative birth movement does not always capture the full complexity of this issue, its proponents have raised vital questions that had been largely ignored in standard obstetric practice.

DISSATISFACTIONS WITH HOSPITAL BIRTH

The health consumer movement, an outgrowth of increasing public awareness together with the erosion of blind trust in physicians, has brought to light issues of cost and of quality of care in obstetrics as in other areas of medicine. As a result, the concerns discussed above have found expression as dissatisfactions with the standard obstetric offering in hospitals. These concerns are summarized in the following list (adapted from Mehl[4]) of desired features of the birth experience:

- to give birth in a relaxed environment where obstetric medication is not encouraged and where friends, relatives, family, and children can give the laboring woman the support she desires to give birth without analgesia or anesthesia and where the birth experience can become as positive a personal/family psychological event as possible
- to be able to choose who will be present at the delivery and to avoid unfamiliar and nonsupportive attendants, nurses, aides, students, residents, and physicians
- to be attended by supportive women attendants—midwives or physicians—who will remain with the woman throughout her labor and birth
- to be more critical concerning obstetric interventions (e.g., electronic fetal monitoring, fetal scalp sampling, intravenous oxytocin, amniotomy)
- to consider alternatives to invasive intervention (e.g., routine cesarean section of breech infants or after 24 hours of ruptured membranes, or routine induction of labor at 42 weeks of gestation)

- to avoid routine episiotomies and to be attended by an individual knowledgeable of delivery styles that minimize the need for episiotomies and the possibility of being torn
- to labor and deliver in the same room in a comfortable position of the woman's own choosing
- to avoid separation of family members after birth, including father, mother, baby, and other siblings
- to avoid quasi-medical indications of separation and to assume a caretaking role along with the medical staff for sick infants
- to be able to breast-feed immediately and on demand
- to avoid long hospital stays
- to avoid routine preparation and enemas
- to be able to move about during labor and to be able to partake of food and drink
- to deliver (in some cases) in out-of-hospital maternity units or in the home

Many women who wish to exercise these choices have turned to what has been throughout history the normal site for birth and remains so in much of the world even today—the home. Some have had births attended only by relatives and friends. When professional attendants have been chosen, it is with the expectation that midwives or physicians who attend home births will respect family prerogatives in decision making and are sensitized to the need for watchful expectancy in labor. Moreover, families have felt that they keep more control on their own ground, where the attendant is an invited guest. Even aside from specific demands and grievances, these women and their partners believe that it does not make sense to go to an alien setting filled with unfamiliar people—a setting associated with illness and contagion—for what is usually a normal, healthy, joyous event.

CHARACTERISTICS OF THOSE CHOOSING HOME BIRTH

In Hazell's study of 300 planned, elective home births between 1969 and 1973 in northern California (a region associated with countercultural life styles), 90 percent of the families surveyed were found to have

> lived in stereotyped American fashion—single family dwelling, fathers gainfully employed, one or two cars, not a member of an ethnic minority, not on welfare, and no household servants. Typ-

ically, both members of the couple have attended college, but neither has graduated. The fathers' occupations were as varied as violinist . . . to auto mechanic.[5]

A profile of 184 families who planned home births between May 1976 and August 1980 in the authors' practice in the Boston-Cambridge metropolitan area yielded similar findings. There was, for example, a preponderance of nuclear-family households. Approximately 80 percent of the parents were married, the remainder being equally divided between unmarried couples and single-parent households. Among those who provided information on their educational backgrounds, approximately 90 percent of both the women and men had had at least some college-level education. Occupations represented included physicians (one obstetrician, one anesthesiologist), nurses, health planners, medical journalists, liberal arts professors, carpenters, cooks, childbirth educators, graduate students, engineers, and restaurateurs. It is particularly striking that some health care professionals have chosen home birth after observing or participating in hospital births.

According to Warner's[6] criteria for estimating social class on the basis of occupation, about half of these families would rank as upper class. This would not be the case for those in the Boston-Cambridge area whose home births are attended by lay midwives or by family and friends alone (rather than by the physician-midwife teams in the authors' practice). Unlike this latter, less-affluent group, two thirds of the families in the sample studied had private health insurance; one sixth had no insurance, and one sixth were on welfare. Remarkably, a number of families who were members of health maintenance organizations chose to pay out of pocket for a home birth rather than use the personnel and facilities covered by the prepaid plan.

Although a comparative study of families seeking home and hospital births in the authors' practice has not been undertaken, it is our judgment that the two groups are not easily distinguishable along either demographic or attitudinal lines. Like the hospital birth group, the home birth group is not careless about the survival of their offspring. On the contrary, these couples take parenthood seriously, are cognizant of the risks entailed by both the home and hospital options, and are motivated to minimize these risks by obtaining and participating in high-quality prenatal care. They do not spurn hospitals and medical specialists when these are really needed. Their explicit preoccupations are similar to those of the families choosing home birth in northern California: nutrition, ecology, preventive medicine, public health, humanistic psychology, personal responsibility, equal partnership between man and woman, and an awareness of oneself as part of a natural and human environment where one's behavior has consequences extending into the future. These concerns have a countercultural flavor, but (especially on the key dimension of personal versus institutional responsibility for decisions concerning life and health) they reflect the part of the counterculture that expresses something akin to frontier individualism. Furthermore, the value placed on family closeness is very much in the American mainstream.

Nonetheless, it must be emphasized that home birth is not limited to the educated, relatively well-to-do segment of the population represented here. Before its recent revival, home birth was primarily associated with poverty, both in rural areas such as that served by the Frontier Nursing Service, with its excellent outcome record,[7] and in urban areas such as that served by the Chicago Maternity Center[8] (see Chapter 2). Moreover, just as the return to breast-feeding, the earlier adoption of bottle-feeding, and hospital birth itself began with an elite group and then spread throughout the population, a similar pattern may emerge in the case of out-of-hospital birth. As more families who lack economic and educational advantages choose to give birth at home or in freestanding birth centers, the careful screening of clients and the maintenance of a high standard of obstetric skill will be abiding concerns for both lay and professional birth attendants.

MIDWIFERY REDISCOVERED

The role of the midwife—that of women helping women at the time of birth—has spanned all ages, cultures, and regions of the world. Yet the place of the midwife in Western civilization has been an equivocal one.[9] In Europe and America the midwife was caricatured as unclean, disorderly, and ignorant by physicians who in many cases knew less about childbirth than she did. Nonetheless, in recognition of the essential contribution to society made by midwives (particularly in serving the rural and urban poor), provisions for the regulation and training of midwives were established in many parts of continental Europe in the nineteenth century and in England in 1902. Although these laws restricted the practice of midwifery, they did allow it to continue, so that midwives later were able to share in the advances in obstetric knowledge that occurred in the early years of the shift from home to hospital birth. This did not happen in America, where midwifery became a very marginal occupation.

The reestablishment of midwifery in the United States came by way of professional training and certification. After the founding of the Maternity Center Association in New York in 1918 and of the Frontier Nursing

Service in Kentucky in 1925, the first training program for nurse-midwives on the British model was begun in 1932. The American College of Nurse-Midwives (ACNM) was incorporated in 1955, but only in 1971 were nurse-midwives officially recognized as primary birth attendants.

Whereas nurse-midwives have practiced extensively in the hospital setting as well as (in some regions) in the home and (more recently) in freestanding birth centers, the home has been the primary arena of lay midwives. Some of the latter are "granny" midwives, holdovers from earlier in the century. Others are younger women who took up the vocation in a spontaneous response to the home birth movement of the 1970s. With physicians usually unavailable for home births (whether because they were not comfortable practicing noninterventive obstetrics, were not comfortable working in the home, feared professional sanctions, or wished to avoid blame for an unfortunate outcome perceived as unlikely to have occurred in the hospital) and nurse-midwives in many areas restricted to hospital practice, a family having a home birth would seek the help of friends, neighbors, or a sympathetic nurse or childbirth educator. Lay midwives arose from the ranks of women who gave birth at home and the female friends who attended them. Learning in the process of doing (as well as by reading and seeking guidance wherever they could find it), some of these women were "certified" as "the midwife" by an underground community network without necessarily having had any wish to take on this title for themselves. They had simply stepped in to fill a need that the physician would not fill and the nurse-midwife could not fill.

Some women have sought out midwives because only midwives would attend their births in the home. Others have had home births because only in the home could they be attended by midwives. Thus there is an important link, both historically and in contemporary practice, between midwifery and home birth. Two issues currently of concern in the development of midwifery as a profession (and as a cultural force) are (1) how lay midwives can be certified by their peers according to standards that guarantee safety and accountability without compromising the unique character of the midwife's work and (2) how lay and nurse-midwives can make common cause to humanize childbirth practices in any setting. These questions are discussed in Chapter 3.

BIRTH CENTERS, BIRTHING ROOMS, AND THE DEMAND FOR HOME BIRTH

As a by-product both of the economic threat it has posed to obstetricians and hospitals and of the substantial validity of its claims, home birth has helped spawn its own competition in the form of in-hospital "birthing rooms" dedicated to providing family-centered maternity care.[10] It has also inspired freestanding birth centers, such as the Childbearing Center operated by the Maternity Center Association in New York, which at one time had maintained a home birth service.[11] These innovations have undoubtedly answered the needs of some families who might otherwise have chosen home birth. That does not mean, however, that they have made home birth unnecessary. Although the question, "Why home birth?" cannot be answered in the 1980s as it was in 1976, for example, it is still very much worth asking. We will consider here some reasons why home birth remains a reasonable and desirable option for some women and their families and how birth attendants and the medical profession can most constructively respond to this choice.

The Choices for Families

Out-of-hospital birth centers staffed by midwives with physician and hospital backup have combined the noninterventive philosophy of home birth with the efficiency resulting from having staff and equipment concentrated in a single location. The authors enthusiastically support the establishment of such centers as a constructive alternative to hospital birth for low-risk pregnancies. Although institutional and procedural issues specific to the birth center format are not discussed in this book, the treatment of clinical questions in Part II is generally applicable to any out-of-hospital setting and should be useful to attendants working in birth centers as well as in the home.

Still, birth centers do not satisfy all the needs that have been met by home birth. For one thing, there are not enough of them and they do not yet have the geographical distribution necessary to serve all those desiring family-centered, noninterventive maternity care in America. As of July 1983, there were 104 centers with nurse-midwives as the primary birth attendants in the Cooperative Birth Center Network (see Appendix A), although the Network reported an accelerating rate of applications for new centers. (Centers staffed primarily by physicians are omitted from this tally, since some of these accept high-risk as well as low-risk labors and do not follow a noninterventive model.[12]) Second, birth centers operate in the same hostile environment that home birth attendants do. No matter how conclusively the excellent safety records, cost savings, and constructive influence of birth centers are demonstrated, concerted and continuing opposition on the part of influential obstetricians and their professional organizations persists.[13] Given their often uneasy relationships with reluctant sponsoring institutions, birth center personnel, like those in publicly visible home birth services, may find themselves under pressure to deviate from their own principles, as by applying overly stringent criteria for initial screening or transfer to hospital.[14] Although some home birth attendants are able to be less visible and thereby more independent, families considering *either* a home birth or a birth center should find out whether the attendants really do have a noninterventive philosophy and how constrained they are by formal or informal sanctions imposed by medical and legal authorities.

In-hospital birthing rooms and the modifications in hospital procedure that they embody, welcome improvements though they may be, are even less plausibly represented as a completely adequate substitute for home birth. It is essential to distinguish between hospital *policy* and hospital *practice*. Many hospitals have liberalized their policies to satisfy a statistically small minority of knowledgeable consumers. However, the interventive philosophy and habits of staff physicians, the training of residents, and the reward structure of an institution where technical procedures earn profit and time spent is money lost remain the same. The chief beneficiaries of the changes in hospital policy are families whose attendants favor the methods usually associated with home birth, yet also have hospital privileges. These attendants (e.g., a physician-midwife team), taking advantage of the liberalized hospital policies, can attend a woman in labor in a birthing room just as they would in her home.

Women who are not fortunate enough to have attendants such as these can still more readily find a hospital-based obstetrician who will attend a planned "natural" (unmedicated) birth than was the case in 1960 or 1970. The obstetrician's stance toward the woman's labor, however, when not medically interventive, often can be characterized as passive. Rarely do hospital-based obstetricians or obstetric nurses bring to a labor the prior knowledge of the woman and family that home birth attendants make it their business to acquire. Rarely do they "labor sit" as described in Chapter 11. Rarely have they mastered the techniques of perineal care that midwives use in place of routine episiotomy. (Admittedly, these generalizations do not recognize the wide range of individual variations in obstetric practice.)

The male partner and other family members, having gained access to the birthing room, are left to do the labor coaching themselves. (Often they do quite well on their own.) Moreover, the threshold for intervention on the part of the hospital staff is often too low. Although the woman now may have a right to refuse treatment, in practice she and her family will need to be forceful and imaginative to avoid interventions such as induction or epidural analgesia if her labor deviates from textbook standards. Thus, if she cannot bring home birth attendants to the hospital as her advocates, the home birth option may alone meet her needs.

These observations do not imply that the home is intrinsically a better place to give birth than the hospital. The question is not one of *site* but of the attendants' *attitude*. Unfortunately, however, there is still a strong association between site and attitude. What constitutes typical practice in a given hospital can be gauged from the rate of frequency of procedures such as cesarean section (which continues to provoke considerable discussion in the obstetric community).[15] If, to use another example, the episiotomy rate declines from 95 percent to 90 percent, how much progress can be claimed?

If birth centers and hospital birthing rooms were widely available and did reliably offer homelike births, some families who now give birth at home would choose these alternatives instead. Many still would not. Of these, some would have residual concerns about continuity of care and decision-making power. Some would want to save money. Others, in the absence of identified risk factors, simply would see no reason to leave their own homes for what they still would perceive to be a natural rather than a medical event.

A medical student who assisted at a home birth in the authors' practice commented as follows:

> About a week earlier I had observed a delivery attended by the same physician and midwife in a hospital birthing room. It looked the same as what I imagined a home birth to be. The people the woman wanted were there, the people she didn't want were not there, and there was no unsolicited medical intervention. I felt that the spirit of a home birth had been captured in the hospital. I was wrong. From the moment I arrived at the home, I sensed that there was something very, very different about a home birth. I had a feeling of peace in that apartment that I had not had in the hospital. To choose your own foods and furnishings, to know where everything is, to be able to move around the house and take a walk outside, to pack in your whole family, to have friends and neighbors drop in—you'd have to move your whole apartment to the hospital to get that kind of freedom and familiarity there.

The Choices for Attendants, the Medical Profession, and Society

The minimal obligation of professionals toward those who choose home birth is stated by Adamson and Gare: "We believe a more humane and respectful approach to these people, while not sacrificing the individual principles of either physician or consumer, is possible and necessary."[16] This translates into the traditional injunction to physicians: *primum non nocere* (first do no harm). Punitive actions such as the denial of prenatal care or of emergency hospital treatment violate this basic humane precept.

Any further involvement in home birth on the part of a midwife or physician rests on the attendant's judgment concerning the safety of home birth, which is discussed in the following chapter. Attendants who do not believe that home birth is a safe alternative or who are not comfortable working without the technical resources of a hospital at hand should not attend home births. On the other hand, those midwives and physicians who are considering seriously the feasibility of attending home births do so out of a desire to honor the fact of human variation by making available the widest range of options consistent with safety. The home birth attendant is tendered a special invitation to share people's lives at a most deeply revealing moment. Home birth gives the attendant an opportunity not only to work collaboratively with knowledgeable partners but also to participate in an intensely satisfying, life-giving experience that can enlarge the capacities of the family and attendant alike.

If a service such as home birth is greatly desired by portions of the public, if it saves money for health insurance providers, if it appears to be approximately as safe as alternative services, if it is a joy for both the family and the attendant, and if it promises to extend the frontiers of knowledge, then it is in the interest of a free society, as well as of the medical profession, to facilitate its availability. For the medical profession to turn its back on a reasonable consumer demand is only to weaken its own credibility and further undermine the trust that is a necessary condition for good health care. Furthermore, both the profession and society have a positive stake in the acquisition of scientific and practical knowledge through innovation.

Perfect procedures and certainty of outcomes will never be achieved. We hold different pieces of knowledge with varying degrees of assurance, but all knowledge is incomplete and subject to evolution and refinement. Home birth presents what to some is a promise and to others a threat— that of teaching us something we do not yet understand. It is in the interest of all concerned to receive this new knowledge in an open but critical spirit by encouraging a free market in ideas and data along with a free market in the delivery of services. If birth centers and birthing rooms reduce or eliminate the demand for home birth, that is the legitimate operation of a free market. But the existence of birth centers and birthing rooms must not be used to justify the suppression (by the harassment and intimidation[17,18] detailed in Chapter 4) of the very competition that has sparked these positive developments.

NOTES

1. Boston Women's Health Book Collective, *Our Bodies, Ourselves: A Book By and For Women,* rev. ed. (New York: Simon & Schuster, 1983).

2. Suzanne Arms, *Immaculate Deception: A New Look at Women and Childbirth in America* (Boston: Houghton Mifflin, 1975).

3. Doris Haire, *The Cultural Warping of Childbirth* (Madison, Wis.: International Childbirth Education Association Special Report, 1972).

4. Lewis E. Mehl, "Options in Maternity Care." Paper presented at the Second Annual Meeting of the National Association of Parents and Professionals for Safe Alternatives in Childbirth, Chicago, Illinois, March 11, 1977.

5. Lester Dessez Hazell, "A Study of 300 Elective Home Births," *Birth and the Family Journal* 2, no. 1 (1975): 11–18.

6. W. Lloyd Warner, with Marchia Meeker and Kenneth Eells, *Social Class in America: A Manual of Procedure for the Measurement of Social Status* (New York: Harper and Brothers, 1960).

7. Eunice K.M. Ernst and Karen A. Gordon, "Fifty-Three Years of Home Birth Experience at the Frontier Nursing Service, Kentucky: 1925–1978," in Lee Stewart and David Stewart, eds., *Compulsory Hospitalization: Freedom of Choice in Childbirth?* (Marble Hill, Mo.: National Association of Parents and Professionals for Safe Alternatives in Childbirth, 1979), vol. 2, pp. 505–516.

8. Margaret Palu et al., "Statistical Outcomes of Elective Home Delivery: II. Comparisons with the Chicago Maternity Center Statistics—Implications for Screening." Paper presented at the International Childbirth Education Association Convention, Seattle, 1976.

9. Fran Ventre and Joan Richards, "The Midwife—Woman With Woman." Unpublished manuscript, Beverly, Mass., 1981.

10. Interprofessional Task Force on Health Care of Women and Children, *Joint Position Statement on the Development of Family-Centered Maternity and Newborn Care in Hospitals* (Chicago, 1978).

11. Jere B. Faison et al., "The Childbearing Center: An Alternative Birth Setting," *Obstetrics and Gynecology* 54 (1979): 527–532.

12. Anita B. Bennetts and Ruth Watson Lubic, "The Free-standing Birth Centre," *Lancet* 1 (1982): 378–380.

13. Wendy Lazarus et al., *Competition Among Health Practitioners: The Influence of the Medical Profession on the Health Manpower Market.* Vol. II: *The Childbearing Center Case Study* (Washington, D.C.: Federal Trade Commission, 1981), p. 33.

14. Ibid., p. 39.

15. Sam Shapiro, Diana Petitti, and Jeanne Guillemin, "The Increase in Cesarean Section Rates: Variations, Risks, and Benefits." Paper presented at the American Public Health Association Meetings, Detroit, Michigan, October 20, 1980.

16. G. David Adamson and Douglas J. Gare, "Home or Hospital Births?" *Journal of the American Medical Association* 243 (1980): 1732–1736.

17. Ilene Tanz Gordon, "The Birth Controllers: Limitations on Out-of-Hospital Births," *Journal of Nurse-Midwifery* 27, no. 1 (January/February 1982): 34–39.

18. Kevin Krajick, "Home vs. Hospital: Where Are Baby, Mother (and Doctor) Safer?" *New Physician,* 31, no. 7 (1982): 14–18.

Chapter 2

The Issue of Safety

Principal Authors: Stanley E. Sagov, M.D., and Archie Brodsky

The fact that home birth has been the norm throughout history and throughout the world is compelling reason to consider this option seriously, but it does not by itself justify home birth as a contemporary practice. Many who are alienated by the medicalization of birth in the United States look to the preservation of a tradition of normal, natural childbirth in many parts of the world as a positive model. In some third-world countries, however, traditional birth practices are associated with rates of fetal and maternal morbidity and mortality that would be unacceptable to Americans. The viability of home birth in America today depends on a discriminating adaptation of historical and cross-cultural experience to modern expectations and standards.

PERCEPTUAL AND INTERPRETIVE BIASES

The prevailing assumption that home birth is not safe is maintained with such apparent inflexibility by the medical profession as well as by substantial segments of American society that it is sometimes impossible even to gain a hearing for an opposing point of view. The orthodoxy reflects an anxious view of birth itself as a treacherous course mined with sudden, unexpected disasters requiring the medical equivalent of a constant military alert. One can most effectively challenge this view by recognizing the reasons—some quite valid when seen from a certain perspective, some not so valid—why so many observers have come to hold it. Although economic interests play a regrettable part in the opposition to home birth, many obstetricians and other physicians genuinely believe that home birth (indeed, any out-of-hospital birth) is dangerous. They do so because they look at it from a different perspective than its proponents do. Demonstrating the safety of home birth is, therefore, partly a matter of showing that one can look at the phenomenon from a different angle.

17

The Historical Bias

In the United States at the turn of the century, hospital birth was generally limited to charity cases and was widely regarded as dangerous. Over the next six decades women in America came to believe that the hospital was a better place to give birth than the home, and yet, according to Devitt,[1] there is no evidence that hospital birth was at any given time safer than home birth for the average woman. Reviewing available data for the period from 1930 to 1960, when there were still enough home births to allow for statistical comparisons (although not conclusive ones), Devitt finds that outcomes were no better in the hospital than in the home. Although poverty and relatively unsanitary conditions were by then associated with the home rather than the hospital, these factors were more than offset by injuries and deaths resulting from obstetric interventions in hospitals. In a famous study of maternal mortality in New York City from 1930 to 1932, conducted by the New York Academy of Medicine, maternal mortality from septicemia, from hemorrhage, and from all causes was significantly lower at home than in the hospital. The difference in mortality rates, which was too pronounced to be explained by the greater proportion of complicated cases delivered in hospitals, was attributed to unnecessary operative interference. The study committee concluded: "It would seem that the present attitude toward home confinements requires re-examination, and a program looking toward an increase in the practice of domiciliary obstetrics deserves careful investigation."[2]

The shift from home to hospital birth in the twentieth century coincided with an impressive reduction in fetal and maternal morbidity and mortality. The advances in obstetric knowledge, practice, and safety that occurred during these years can, however, be understood in terms of factors other than site, such as improved nutrition, lower birth rates, fewer low-birth-weight babies, fewer closely spaced children, fewer instances of grand multiparity, the availability of antibiotics, better detection of disorders such as toxemia of pregnancy and anemia, and more accurate risk assessment through antenatal fetal monitoring, ultrasound, amniocentesis, routine serologies, and the availability of blood and blood products.[3-7] Some of these developments represented improvements in public health resulting from demographic and social change rather than from the site of birth; some reflected increased awareness among professionals and the public (awareness that was more effectively transmitted in the hospital setting); some resulted from research made possible by the centralization and standardization of birth in the hospital; some involved equipment that initially could not be used outside the hospital.

It is likely, then, that the transition from home to hospital had an important although indirect effect on the improvement of obstetric outcomes in the twentieth century, primarily (perhaps exclusively) through the detection and management of complications of labor and delivery. It is, in fact, this very codification of information and refinement of procedures that now gives birth attendants the freedom to decentralize, to be less bound by site and more attentive to human as opposed to technical concerns. With the miniaturization of technology (e.g., portable ultrasound monitors) and the availability of antibiotics, aseptic technique, competent midwives and physicians, good prenatal care outside the hospital, and mobile flying-squad "operating room" ambulances along with regular ambulance transport, the hospital site need no longer be a prerequisite to reasonable assurance of a safe outcome.

This is not, however, how the situation has been perceived. During the decades of transition, when hospital birth attracted the most knowledgeable physicians and the most healthy, well-informed, and well-to-do women, a de facto association developed between home birth and poverty, ignorance, malnutrition, and consequent bad outcomes. This association was an artifact of history. Nonetheless, in a classic example of what cognitive psychologists call *illusory correlation*,[8] it has been taken to represent an actual (and unchanging) cause-and-effect relationship. The obstetricians who have engendered the current climate of hostility toward home birth were trained at a time when home birth might reasonably have been seen as more dangerous than hospital birth. Their attitude is understandable in the light of their formative professional experiences. A new generation of obstetricians has in some instances been able to disentangle the illusory correlation and take a fresh look at the changing relationship between site and safety. But their training, too, has reflected the preconceptions of their elders.

The Consultant's Perspective

A specialist who receives referrals of complicated cases may never see firsthand how few in proportion to the total those cases actually are. An intern who sutures severe perineal tears in the emergency room may understandably believe that failure to perform an episiotomy has dire consequences, since the many women who forgo episiotomy without significant perineal tears never reach the emergency room. Similarly, an obstetric consultant whose only contact with home birth comes from seeing complicated cases arrive at the hospital is unlikely to rhapsodize over the beauty of normal labor in the home. The selection bias that operates here is unfortunate. People who are positioned so as to see only the occasional bad outcome assume the bad outcome to be the rule.

Idealized View of the Hospital

Those who reject home birth as dangerous often judge it against an assumed standard of certainty and perfection that is identified with the hospital. One does not have to slight the high quality of care that many American hospitals seek to provide in the 1980s to realize, on reflection, that the assumed standard is an unrealistic one. Advocates of out-of-hospital birth point to the iatrogenic complications that have been shown to result from obstetric intervention not only in the older studies cited above but also in more recent ones.[9] Some observers believe that the availability and profitability of interventive technology in hospitals motivate its inappropriate as well as appropriate use and that one intervention risks touching off a chain of further interventions.[10] Another form of iatrogenesis observed in the authors' clinical experience is that which is unwittingly introduced by overworked staff members whose judgment is impaired by fatigue and whose working conditions preclude their getting to know clients and identifying with their interests.[11] (The effects of overwork are also felt by home birth services in areas where punitive actions against home birth attendants cause too great a demand to be placed on the few physicians and midwives willing to attend home births, who may then be unable to provide the quality of personal care that home birth requires.)

Even aside from the issue of iatrogenesis, the assumption that adequate provision for emergencies is ensured by the mere choice of the hospital setting does not fit the facts. Hospitals vary greatly with respect to the availability of personnel and equipment in readiness for rare, unpredictable, potentially dangerous events. These variations are recognized in proposals for regionalization of maternity care services, which use risk-factor protocols for assigning cases to primary, secondary, or tertiary care centers.[12] Such plans systematize the triage decisions that are routinely made regarding whether a birth should take place in one hospital or another and when a consultation or transfer between hospitals is indicated. For example, a newborn at high risk may be transferred from a community hospital to a neonatal intensive-care unit in a tertiary care center. Thus, the risk assessment procedures outlined in this book for home birth screening and transfer to hospital represent clinical and policy judgments of the same order as those made—with less controversy—within the hospital framework. Unexpected, life-threatening emergencies do very occasionally occur in the home. But some of the hospitals in which these occur are hardly better staffed and equipped to deal with them than a home or birth center would be. These rare emergencies are unavoidable because human beings cannot predict the future with absolute certainty and because society cannot afford the costs, human and monetary, of having every baby born in a high-risk, maximal-technology center.

No clinician and no institution can be perfectly prepared for every eventuality, particularly when more than one crisis can occur at the same time. Although hospitals as a rule offer more ready access to specialized personnel and facilities than do out-of-hospital sites, an immediate response to an emergency is not guaranteed even in the hospital. It may take some time, for example, to assemble the equipment, space, and on-call personnel needed to perform a cesarean section. Thus, the 10 or 20 minutes spent transporting a woman in labor from her home or a freestanding birth center to the hospital (if preceded by a telephone call preparing the hospital staff for the patient's arrival and clinical needs) may in practice be equivalent to the time it can take to move a woman from an in-hospital birthing room to an operating room. Indeed, many community hospitals without full-time obstetric staff do not even have the capacity for immediate cesarean sections.

Misconceptions about Science

Conceptions of science and of scientific practice are important to the debate on home birth in at least two ways. First, the data on outcomes of home and hospital birth must be evaluated by criteria for validity in scientific investigation. Second, opponents of home birth (e.g., the Executive Director of the American College of Obstetricians and Gynecologists in a 1977 newsletter) have characterized people who have home births as being in revolt against science and against intellect.[13] The practice of obstetricians in hospitals is identified with science, while that of home birth attendants is portrayed as primitive, obscurantist, and Luddite. At the core of the case for home birth, then, is a demonstration that the procedures of responsible home birth attendants, even though they do not fit the image of the white-coated laboratory technician, are deeply reflective of contemporary scientific principles.

Certainty through Technology

The image of science against which home birth is found wanting is one in which the goal is certainty; the means, technology. All possible information is sought in an effort to remove uncertainty, doubt, and surprise—aims that are so urgent psychologically that the costs of obtaining the information may not be considered. Moreover, the ritualized use of technological means can become so reassuring and thereby rewarding in itself that it is perpetuated irrespective of whether ends (diagnostic or therapeutic) are being met. In this way both costs and benefits are obscured by an illusory correlation—that between the application of technology and the acquisition of useful knowledge.[14,15] Although this uncritical enthusiasm for technology is found in all branches of medicine, it was given special impetus in obstetrics in the early decades of this century by the denigration of obstetricians as being less skilled than more actively interventive physicians in other specialties. As Devitt[16] observes, if the obstetrician wanted to be recognized as a true scientist, the model held out for emulation was that of the surgeon.

The uncritical use of technology in obstetrics is exemplified by electronic fetal monitoring (EFM).[17] EFM is of demonstrated value in the management of complicated labors, but its value (compared with that of careful auscultation) in uncomplicated labors and the frequency and severity of its alleged side effects (an increased rate of cesarean sections and a slight risk of infection and of injury to the fetus) remain a matter of debate.[18–23] Nonetheless, EFM has been adopted for routine and costly use in hospital obstetrics. In 1978 it was estimated that EFM was used in two thirds of all births in the United States.[24] According to a study conducted at the Harvard School of Public Health, this new technology was disseminated so rapidly that many physicians may have come to use it without having learned to interpret which of the abnormalities revealed by the monitor require intervention. Ironically, the accumulation of diagnostic data (some of it artifactual) in the service of "defensive medicine" has created a need for defensive treatment. Once even an insignificant deviation from the norm is recorded on a tracing that becomes a permanent part of the record, the physician feels legally vulnerable if he or she fails to intervene. As one of the Harvard investigators was quoted as saying, "It is possible for better information to change treatment decisions for the worse."[25]

The Harvard study concludes that large areas of uncertainty remain concerning the appropriate use of EFM. Obstetricians have become more discriminating in their identification of abnormal readings that constitute indications for intervention. The use of fetal scalp sampling in conjunction with EFM has made the latter a more effective diagnostic tool. At the same time, techniques of auscultation have also been refined. Therefore, prior comparative studies may have limited relevance today, and an openness to new data would appear to be essential. Yet a group of obstetricians interviewed about EFM did not acknowledge this uncertainty. Instead, they expressed attitudes of strong acceptance (four fifths) or strong rejection (one fifth).[26] As a result, those who do not use EFM in low-risk labors are placed in the position of having to defend this choice, and the lack of EFM (even in a screened low-risk population) is cited as a disadvantage of home birth. For those who believe that it is a disadvantage, a portable fetal monitor that can be taken to the home is available. For the above reasons, however, the authors do not recommend its use.

Contemporary Scientific Standards

Automatic technological intervention, a function of deterministic thinking and one-dimensional decision making, is scientific only in a mechanistic, eighteenth-century sense. Twentieth-century science, in particular physics, provides a probabilistic model for medical research and practice. Bursztajn and associates[27] outline the basic principles of probabilistic science and their application to clinical decision making. These involve a recognition of multicausality (with causes being in flux and not absolutely knowable), of the effects of the observer on the observed (e.g., the effects of the physician-patient relationship on the course of illness), and of the scientific validity and usefulness of subjective ("soft") data and its interrelatedness with objective ("hard") data.

This modern view of science is grounded in an awareness of uncertainty as an ever-present fact of existence. It does not, however, give license for carelessness, wishful thinking, mysticism, or inexactitude in clinical investigation. On the contrary, it challenges the physician or midwife to a comprehensive assessment of more subtle forms of data and more subtle relationships among variables than the mechanistic model allows for. Judgments are based on a range of information, some of which is less easy to measure than a fetal heart rate. For example, the incidence of some complications of labor has been found to be affected by psychological factors.[28] Some women may react to the stresses of the hospital environment by developing tensions that in turn complicate labor and may therefore require medical interventions that would not have been required in what for them is the more tranquil, confidence-inspiring setting of their own homes. Others, who have stressful home environments, may experience less anxiety in the hospital.

Bursztajn and associates use a home birth as a case example of contemporary scientific method.[29] Elements of a well-planned home birth that illustrate important features of probabilistic decision making include individualized management, emphasis on choice rather than determinacy, dynamic assessment of risks and benefits, and attention to values along with probabilities. The combination of objective and subjective information that a home birth attendant acquires prenatally through careful screening and personal contact becomes the basis for sensitive probability estimates during labor. When a woman has an arrest of dilatation, an attendant who has come to know the woman well may be able to choose with some confidence between two interpretations: "Arrest of labor—suspected cephalopelvic disproportion," or "This woman is emotionally blocked about having her baby." Such interpretation is not just intuition. It is a Bayesian estimate, based on prior probabilities, of the probability that a given clinical sign has one meaning as opposed to another.[30] Family members present at a birth can also provide clinically useful information. For example, if progress is slow and the baby's position is posterior, testimony from the laboring woman's mother that her own labors had progressed well after spontaneous rotation to the anterior position should carry a degree of reassurance. Such information can be used in hospital as well as home births, but hospital birth attendants are less likely to avail themselves of it, perhaps because they place such great confidence in the technology at hand. Their confidence may not always be warranted, just as some home birth attendants may place unwarranted confidence in personal, subjective knowledge when technology is needed.

OUTCOMES OF HOME AND HOSPITAL BIRTHS

The preceding commentary is intended to provide a framework for understanding the data that follow. These data are taken from historical and cross-cultural studies as well as from comparisons of outcomes of home and hospital births within the same country at the same time, although only in the Netherlands among industrialized countries are there currently enough home births to make meaningful comparisons of this last sort.

European and Cross-Cultural Data

In Great Britain there has been a dramatic shift from predominantly home to predominantly hospital delivery since 1958. The benefits of hospital care are said to be reflected in the fact that the overall stillbirth rate in England and Wales has fallen in recent years while the stillbirth rate for home delivery infants has not.[31] However, this phenomenon may be due both to the greater number of uncomplicated deliveries now taking place in the hospital and to improved methods of treating the complicated conditions that occur among hospital births. The perinatal mortality rate among low-risk births in the home may, on the other hand, already have been at a low baseline (4.9 per thousand in 1970) that has remained difficult to improve on.

Other British studies cast considerable doubt on whether increased hospitalization has brought about improved outcomes. In Cardiff, Wales, a shift from predominantly home to hospital deliveries between 1965 and 1973 has had essentially no effect on maternal or neonatal outcomes.[32] Perinatal mortality rates in England were lower in local authorities with higher rates of hospital confinement until 1967, after which the trend was reversed.[33] Tew,[34] surveying maternal and neonatal outcomes between 1965 and 1974, found no evidence, even after correcting for the higher concentration of risk factors in hospital births, that the move from home to hospital had brought about a decrease in the perinatal mortality rate. In response to these data and to consumer demand, there has been a small swing back to home birth in Great Britain.[35]

The best natural laboratory for home birth outcome research is in the Netherlands, where national policy, a noninterventive philosophy of birth, and an excellent support system have enabled midwives and general practitioners to continue to attend almost half of the nation's births at home. Kloosterman,[36] analyzing data compiled by the Central Bureau of Statistics, finds no significant differences in outcomes between cities with almost 100 percent of births in the hospital and cities of similar demography with only a 50 percent rate of hospital births (although there is more obstetric intervention in the hospital). Cross-cultural comparisons between the Netherlands and other Western European countries such as Great Britain, West Germany, and Sweden, where virtually all births are in the hospital, also show no significant differences in outcomes.

Between 1960 and 1977 the proportion of deliveries in the Netherlands occurring in the home declined from 70 percent to 40 percent.[37] Some observers attribute the decreasing perinatal mortality rate in Holland to this change.[38] However, the rate has actually declined in both settings— from 60.0 to 22.7 per thousand in the hospital and from 14.0 to 4.2 per thousand at home between 1960 and 1974.[39] (The higher figures for the hospital are a function of complicated, including preterm, deliveries and should not in themselves be taken to favor home birth.) As in other Western industrialized countries, these improvements are attributable primarily to advances in public health, secondarily to improved prenatal and postnatal care, and only slightly to improved perinatal care. Supporting this conclusion with a range of data, Kloosterman[40] points out, for example, that perinatal mortality due to anencephaly (a congenital anomaly incompatible with life, unrelated to place or manner of birth, and readily diagnosed even without today's highly developed diagnostic skills) has decreased slightly more than has total perinatal mortality.

Further refutation of the alleged link between increased hospitalization and improved outcomes is provided by a study in which 3,000 women in a small Dutch city were screened for perinatal risk. Eighty percent of these women were found eligible to give birth at home and did so with a very

low perinatal mortality rate of 2.5 per thousand.[41] North American physicians have speculated that such results are made possible by a homo-
geneous population of women whose bodies are optimally proportioned
for childbearing. According to Kloosterman, however, demographic shifts
have created in the Netherlands a mixed population without bringing about
a worsening of perinatal statistics.[42] Devitt[43] compared outcomes of birth
in the Netherlands in 1972 with those in the demographically similar (e.g.,
in population density) state of Massachusetts. Even with the black population eliminated from the Massachusetts figures, the Netherlands had a
lower infant mortality rate with less investment in physicians and hospital
facilities but greater investment in home maternity aides.

Home birth in the Netherlands has a beneficial effect on that nation's
entire system of obstetric care. Through the repeated experience and
highly visible model of successful normal births in the home, as well as
through the prominent role of midwives in hospitals as well as at home, a
noninterventive philosophy of maternity care (relative to other countries)
is maintained even for hospital births.[44,45] The incidence of cesarean section
in the Netherlands was 2.0 percent in 1969, 3.0 percent in 1975, and 5.0
percent in 1980. In the United States the rate was 5.3 percent in 1969, 10.2
percent in 1975, and 15.2 percent in 1978. Although the rate of instrumental
deliveries in the United States is declining as that of cesarean sections
rises, in 1975 it was still 33.5 percent as compared with 4.9 percent in the
Netherlands.[46–48]

The data from the Netherlands, Great Britain, and other European
countries suggest that site is not a decisive factor in the outcome of birth.
Studies comparing outcomes in America with those in countries such as
Norway and Sweden, which also have virtually 100 percent hospitalization
for birth yet have much lower perinatal mortality rates, have identified
what does seem to be the most decisive factor: birth weight.[49,50] The best
hope for reducing perinatal mortality in the United States lies in reducing
the proportion of low-birth-weight, high-risk infants. This conclusion is
echoed even in American studies of the beneficial effects of obstetric
interventions.[51] Seen in this light, the controversy about site is a diversion
from the real issue of prenatal prevention and/or identification of preterm
and other low-birth-weight deliveries.

American Data

Data on out-of-hospital birth in the United States are available not only
for home birth but also for freestanding birth centers such as that run by
the Maternity Center Association of New York (which previously had
operated a home birth service, with nurse-midwives in attendance, that

achieved neonatal and maternal mortality rates considerably lower than the local and national averages for the time[52]). A report prepared for the Federal Trade Commission concluded that during its first five years of operation (1975–1980) the association's Childbearing Center had maintained a high standard of safety and offered high-quality care at low cost, while exerting a positive influence on obstetric care in the New York area and nationally.[53] A 1982 study of almost 2,000 labors in 11 such centers, each staffed by nurse-midwives with a noninterventive philosophy, yielded similar findings. Of the women who began labor at the centers, 5 percent had instrumental deliveries and 5 percent had cesarean sections at a backup hospital. Apgar scores of 7 to 10 were recorded for 93 percent of the infants at one minute and for 95 percent at five minutes. The neonatal death rate was 4.6 per thousand live births including transfers and 3.0 per thousand excluding transfers.[54]

A freestanding birth center is essentially equivalent to a home birth service in which well-trained personnel follow the screening and clinical procedures outlined in Part II of this book. With respect to safety, a birth center offers prospective clients the advantage of an established institutional reputation, so that families are spared the necessity of evaluating the credentials of the individual attendants. (A birth center—or, for that matter, a home birth service—may, however, be run like a physicians' group practice with rotating calls and may therefore not provide the personal care traditionally associated with midwives.) The birth center may also have marginal advantages with respect to routinized procedures and a physical layout set up for the convenience and familiarity of the attendants. However, since the center is not equipped for maximally interventive responses to obstetric emergencies, its clinical protocols, including those pertaining to transfer to hospital, must be approximately the same as those observed in the home. It is reasonable to expect, then, that competently managed home birth services can duplicate the impressive safety record of the birth centers in the study cited above.

A highly successful example of a home birth service in America is that of the Frontier Nursing Service in Kentucky. The people it has served since 1925 are not ideal candidates for home birth, since they tend to be geographically remote, inbred, impoverished, and undereducated. Yet the service, whose nurse-midwives attended nearly all births at home until the late 1960s, has had fetal, infant, and maternal mortality and morbidity rates that compare favorably with those of middle-class America.[55] Beginning in 1953 the Frontier Nursing Service has compiled a record of more than 10,000 births over a quarter of a century without a maternal death. According to preliminary indications, however, the recent increase in hospital deliveries by the service (due to Medicaid eligibility) has been

associated with increased rates of intervention but no significant improvement in outcomes.[56]

A less successful example was that of the Chicago Maternity Center,
which served a comparably poor urban population that lacked adequate
childbirth education. Although on balance the center served this community well (its closing in the mid 1970s was bitterly protested), its home
deliveries resulted in higher neonatal mortality rates and greater neurological abnormality and fetal hypoxia than in other home or hospital birth
samples studied in the same period. These outcomes were associated with
the use of anesthesia, analgesia, intravenous oxytocin, and forceps delivery in the home.[57] They were a reflection not on home birth, but on an
inappropriate match between site and techniques. The useful lesson learned
from the Chicago Maternity Center experience is that hospitallike obstetric
interventions in the home are not a satisfactory substitute for good prenatal
care, a noninterventive approach, and timely transfer to hospital.

In Mehl and associates'[58] well-known matched comparison study, completed in 1976, 1,046 women who planned a home birth (including 12
percent who transferred to hospitals during labor) were individually matched
against an equal number of women who planned to deliver in a hospital.
They were matched for maternal age, parity, educational level, socioeconomic status, length of gestation, and risk factor score prior to the incep-
tion of labor. There were no significant differences between the two groups
in birth weight or in perinatal mortality, neurological abnormalities, or
other major complications. However, almost every type of obstetric intervention (including oxytocin, episiotomy, forceps delivery, cesarean section, and local, regional, and general anesthesia) was employed more
frequently in the planned hospital births. The latter also showed a significantly higher rate of complications, such as third- and fourth-degree perineal tears (even with more episiotomies), fetal distress, hypertension and
preeclampsia, shoulder dystocia, postpartum hemorrhage, respiratory distress syndrome, birth injuries, and neonatal sepsis. Overall, the planned
hospital births showed a higher resuscitation rate and more noncongenital
neonatal complications than the planned home births. The latter group
showed greater intrapartum bleeding and more cases of posterior delivery
(accepted as a normal variant by home birth attendants) and second-stage
dystocia. The study (which should not in itself be taken as authoritative,
since the data collection and matching were not reviewed by a refereed
journal) raised serious questions about obstetric iatrogenesis. However,
subsequent review and modification of hospital procedures would likely
reduce the observed differences between the home and hospital groups if
the study were to be repeated now.

Estes'[59] study of outcomes in his home birth service in Mill Valley, California, between 1974 and 1977 (which is also an excellent summary of the screening criteria, equipment, and backup procedures employed by a well-run service) reported on 418 planned home births, including 49 antepartum transfers, 19 hospitalizations for premature labor, 61 intrapartum transfers, and 289 completed home births. The overall stillbirth rate was 4.72 per thousand; the stillbirth rate in the home was 3.47 per thousand. The uncorrected overall perinatal mortality rate was 16.28 per thousand; when corrected for major congenital anomalies incompatible with life, the rate was 9.45 per thousand. At home the perinatal death rate was 10.31 per thousand uncorrected and 3.47 per thousand corrected. Neonatal mortality at home was 8.77 per thousand uncorrected and zero per thousand corrected. There were no maternal deaths. The outcomes for this small sample of carefully planned and attended home births were comparable to those for low-risk hospital births.

Other studies have focused on the different types of practitioners, particularly unlicensed lay midwives, involved in home birth. A matched comparison of 421 home births attended by noncertified midwives judged by the investigators to be experienced and knowledgeable with an equal number of hospital births attended by physicians yielded better outcomes for the midwives. When only the less interventionist half of the physicians were compared with the midwives, few significant differences were found.[60] An analysis of all out-of-hospital births recorded in Oregon in 1977 found that while 19 percent of unlicensed attendants reported births with no prenatal care, a majority of these were fathers and fellow members of religious communities. All of the clients of lay midwives had prenatal care, with 71 percent beginning in the first trimester. The neonatal and infant death rates for out-of-hospital births were lower than those for all births in Oregon and in the United States in the same year, while the incidence of full-term fetal deaths, although twice as high as that for all full-term births in Oregon, was still a relatively low 6.0 per thousand.[61] These outcomes were encouraging, especially in view of the inclusion of births attended by unlicensed and in some cases unskilled attendants.

Raw statewide perinatal mortality statistics such as these have been used in a misleading way to discredit home birth, most notably in a 1978 news release by the American College of Obstetricians and Gynecologists (ACOG), which claimed, on the basis of data from 11 state health departments, that the risk to a baby's life was two to five times greater in an out-of-hospital birth than a hospital birth.[62] The media exposure given this announcement was undeserved and unfortunate, since the conclusion drawn was based on a misinterpretation of the data. Lumped together in the "out-of-hospital" category, along with elective home births, were many late miscarriages, premature and precipitous (i.e., unplanned) deliveries, and unattended home births. In California, for example, birth-weight statistics indicate that two thirds of the out-of-hospital deaths were premature deliveries.[63]

As a corrective to such misuse of data, a major study of home births in North Carolina during 1974 through 1976, conducted by the Center for Disease Control in Atlanta, demonstrated the importance of eliminating confounding variables in comparisons between sites. This study concluded that "deliveries occurring at home ranged from lowest to highest risk of neonatal mortality depending on planning and the attendant present." Neonatal mortality rates were 3 per thousand live births for planned home births attended by a lay midwife, 30 per thousand for planned home births without a lay midwife, and 120 per thousand for unplanned home births.[64]

The authors have pooled their data from a family practice in Cambridge, Massachusetts, with data obtained by two physicians in Fresno, California, whose practice employs screening protocols very similar to the authors'. The total number of women seeking home births in the two practices between 1976 and 1982 was 875. Data on transfers and outcomes for this sample are presented in Table 2-1. (Transfer statistics are further broken down according to indications for transfer in Tables 2-2 through 2-4, which appear in Appendix 2-A.) The overall picture is an encouraging one, with no maternal deaths, modest rates of transfer and intervention, and few major complications. Birth weight clustered in the 3,000 to 4,000 gram range, with 14 infants below 2,500 grams among the antepartum transfers and 9 among the 727 labors begun at home. Most of the infants born at home had Apgar scores (a less objective measure) of 8 to 10 at one minute (85.2 percent) and at five minutes (97.3 percent).

However, the stillbirth rate of 8.25 per thousand labors begun at home is higher than in other studies. Three of the six stillbirths, antepartum fetal deaths discovered in early labor (having occurred after the last prenatal examination from one day to one week earlier), took place within one four-month period in the California practice. The stillbirth rate is declining as more births are added. The three deaths, along with a similar fatality in the Massachusetts sample, had occurred by the time the birth attendant arrived (without delay) at the home (and presumably, then, before the woman would have chosen to go to the hospital had she planned to deliver there). In one case vasa previa was identified as a probable cause. No cause was established in the other three cases (in two of which autopsy was refused). Precipitate labor appears to have been a factor in two of these deaths. All four are judged not to have been site related or preventable.

Table 2-1 Outcomes of Planned Home Births

	Number	Rate per 1,000 labors begun at home
Total seeking home birth	875	
Lost to follow-up	69	
(moved, transferred)		
Continued prenatal care	806	
Changed to planned hospital in antepartum	79	
Began labor at home	727	
Intrapartum transfers	56	
Postpartum transfers	17	
Maternal	10	
Neonatal	7	
Planned and completed without transfer	654	
Home births	671	
Stillbirths (see text)	6*	8.25
Antepartum	4	5.50
Intrapartum	2	2.75
Live home births	666	
Cesarean sections	22	30.26 (3.0%)
Maternal deaths	0	

*One stillbirth occurred in hospital.

Source: Family Practice Group, Cambridge, Massachusetts, and David Dowis, M.D. and Janet Dowis, M.D., Fresno, California.

A fifth stillbirth occurred after a 43.5-week gestation in early active labor in the home while normal protocols for auscultation were being followed. Postterm antenatal screening (urine estriol determinations and nonstress tests) failed to predict fetoplacental insufficiency. Although by our revised protocol this birth would have occurred in the hospital, the literature and clinical experience do not support the contention that EFM would have reliably prevented the stillbirth, which therefore cannot be said to be site related. To have intervened to prevent this prolonged gestation by prior induction would have raised questions regarding the costs and benefits of such a policy for all affected cases.

The other stillbirth occurred in a primigravid breech birth after extensive counseling in which the attendants explained the risks and advised in favor of a hospital birth. When the couple, duly informed, announced their intention to deliver at home with or without professional assistance, the attendants agreed to attend the birth. In the presence of two physicians and two nurses (one a neonatal intensive-care nurse), a stillborn infant was delivered within nine minutes after fetal heart tones were last auscultated. Resuscitation (including confirmed endotracheal intubation) was initiated immediately without success. On examination Potter's syndrome was suspected, but autopsy was refused. Since EFM or elective cesarean section might have altered the outcome, this death may be regarded as possibly site related—an eventuality anticipated by the attendants when they strongly recommended hospital delivery. Overall, only two of the six stillbirths in our series may have been site related.

. Studies in two leading academic centers in Boston have shown that perinatal death rates for term infants can be reduced to very low levels—in one study 1 per thousand low-risk newborns,[65] in the other study 0.43 per thousand intrapartum (along with 1.79 per thousand antepartum and 1.3 per thousand neonatal) for all term infants.[66] In the second study the combined intrapartum and neonatal death rate for normally formed term infants was approximately 1 per thousand. These outcomes, achieved in two of the finest obstetric departments in the world, cannot be taken as representative of the hospital site generally, nor are they directly comparable with the home birth data reported here, since the study populations are not numerically equal and were not matched for comparison. It is, however, worth noting that, with four of the six stillbirths in our sample classified as antepartum (since the fetal heart was not heard in labor despite the attendants' prompt response), the intrapartum stillbirth rate for this home birth sample was just 2.75 per thousand.

The prospect of the virtual elimination of perinatal mortality in uncomplicated labors (in the absence of lethal congenital malformations) is to be welcomed. Just as home birth can be seen as a laboratory for exploring the potency of natural processes and thereby humanizing hospital obstetrics, so there is much in the triumphs of hospital obstetrics that can be usefully adapted to out-of-hospital sites. As the advancement and exchange of knowledge in the two sites proceeds, however, it is hoped that fetal and neonatal mortality rates will be evaluated in a larger context that also includes consideration of fetal and maternal morbidity and of the long-term viability of infants whose lives are saved by heroic means.

INTERPRETATION OF THE DATA

Historical, cross-cultural, observational, and matched comparison studies yield reassuring findings about the safety of birth both in and out of hospitals. Nature has endowed human reproduction with favorable chances of success. Good prenatal care enhances these prospects and allows for identification of most births that will require more than minimal technical intervention. Competent attendants and appropriate use of technology at birth further improve the odds of a positive outcome. Differences in safety between the home and hospital sites appear to be statistically marginal and in certain respects may favor the home as well as the hospital. Nonetheless, any unnecessary loss of life is cause for deep concern and raises ethical issues for all those involved.

Adamson and Gare's[67] balanced review of the literature on home versus hospital birth is a corrective to impassioned partisanship on both sides and a good starting point for an assessment of risks. It cites unanticipated complications that can cause severe morbidity or mortality unless treated quickly and effectively. Most of the treatments required are, however, site independent, although some require special skills of the attendants. Laceration, retained placenta, and uterine inversion can be treated out of hospital depending on the expertise and equipment available. The "ABCs" of resuscitation are easily performed in the home, as is intubation to allow for suction of meconium or other aspiration (see Chapter 12). Oxygen can be brought to the home and can be used together with intravenous fluid support in treatment for shock. Even cord prolapse, for which prompt cesarean section is indicated, involves gradations of risk, since mothers and infants have (with proper positioning) survived for hours during transport from outlying regions. Nonetheless, there is a very slight possibility that a complication such as placenta accreta (which requires emergency hysterectomy) could, in the absence of an obstetric flying squad, result in a site-related death out of hospital or in a hospital not staffed and equipped for a prompt surgical response. However, the determination of the level of incidence of such rare calamities that should trigger large-scale policy decisions affecting all births is not simply a medical decision (in the narrow sense) but a moral and political decision involving technical, monetary, and ethical considerations.

The authors' clinical experience supports Kloosterman's[68] estimate that for a well-screened low-risk population the probability of an emergent complication (e.g., fetal distress, severe postpartum hemorrhage), which would make the loss of time in transit to hospital a serious disadvantage in managing the labor (whether or not it results in a bad outcome), is less than one per thousand. Families must be informed of this very small but real risk, which they must balance against the risks, largely iatrogenic and psychological, incurred in the hospital. Whether a family chooses to take the risk and whether society chooses to regard it as a legitimate one are cost-benefit decisions (the benefits being those described in Chapter 1). They are no different from other clinical decisions (ranging from routine laboratory tests and prescriptions to life-and-death questions of treatment for heart disease or cancer) that are made by weighing the probabilities of different outcomes along with the values attached to those outcomes. With respect to home birth the values at stake are outlined in the previous chapter, the probabilities, in this chapter. In a society where large risks are taken for granted in connection with activities such as automobile travel, consumption of alcohol and tobacco, and dangerous sports—a society where, for example, pregnant women are not legally required to wear seat belts in automobiles—the small risks of home birth do not seem unreasonable ones to incur in return for the benefits of enhanced psychological and physiological functioning and family integrity.

Citizens and professionals who are troubled by the risks can contribute constructively in two ways: first, by facilitating the collection of more and better data about home birth, and second, by helping to create support systems that will reduce the already minimal risks of home birth. As things stand, home birth attendants are stuck on the horns of a dilemma poignantly described in the Federal Trade Commission report on the Maternity Center Association's Childbearing Center: "the two doctors who claimed that positive data could convince them of the Center's adequacy were vehemently opposed to the operation of the Center. Therefore, their claim that they could be persuaded to change their opinions appears illusory, as data collection in the absence of services is an impossibility."[69]

NOTES

1. Neal Devitt, "The Transition from Home to Hospital Birth in the United States, 1930–1960," *Birth and the Family Journal* 4 (1977): 47–58.

2. Ibid., p. 53.

3. Dugald Baird, "The Obstetrician and Society," *American Journal of Public Health* 60 (1970): 628–640.

4. Iain Chalmers, J.G. Lawson, and A.C. Turnbull, "Evaluation of Different Approaches to Obstetric Care," *British Journal of Obstetrics and Gynaecology* 83 (1976): 921–933.

5. E. Stewart Taylor, "Determinants of the Neonatal Mortality " (editorial comment), *Obstetrical and Gynecological Survey* 32 (1977): 153–155.

6. J.R. Ashford, "Policies for Maternity Care in England and Wales: Too Fast and Too Far?" in Sheila Kitzinger and John A. Davis (eds.), *The Place of Birth* (New York: Oxford University Press, 1978), pp. 14–43.

7. Peter Huntingford, "Obstetric Practice: Past, Present, and Future," in Sheila Kitzinger and John A. Davis (eds.), *The Place of Birth* (New York: Oxford University Press, 1978), pp. 229–250.

8. Richard A. Shweder, "Likeness and Likelihood in Everyday Thought: Magical Thinking and Everyday Judgments about Personality," in P.N. Johnson-Laird and P.C. Wason (eds.), *Thinking: Readings in Cognitive Science* (Cambridge, England: Cambridge University Press, 1977), pp. 446–467.

9. Lewis E. Mehl, "The Outcome of Home Delivery: Research in the United States," in Sheila Kitzinger and John A. Davis (eds.), *The Place of Birth* (New York: Oxford University Press, 1978), pp. 93–117.

10. M.P.M. Richards, "A Place of Safety? An Examination of the Risks of Hospital Delivery," in Sheila Kitzinger and John A. Davis (eds.), *The Place of Birth* (New York: Oxford University Press, 1978), pp. 66–84.

11. Jerry Edelwich with Archie Brodsky, *Burnout: Stages of Disillusionment in the Helping Professions* (New York: Human Sciences Press, 1980), pp. 153–157, 164–167.

12. Committee on Perinatal Health, The National Foundation—March of Dimes, *Toward Improving the Outcome of Pregnancy: Recommendations for the Regional Development of Maternal and Perinatal Health Services* (White Plains, N.Y., 1976).

13. Warren H. Pearse, "Home Birth Crisis," *American College of Obstetricians and Gynecologists Newsletter*, July 1977.

14. Harold Bursztajn, Robert M. Hamm, and Thomas G. Gutheil, "Involving the Patient in Decision Making: Promises and Pitfalls of Formal and Informal Approaches," in Stanley Reiser and Michael Anbar (eds.), *Implementing Medical Technology: Issues and Strategies* (Cambridge, England: Cambridge University Press, in press).

15. Harold Bursztajn et al., *Medical Choices, Medical Chances: How Patients, Families, and Physicians Can Cope With Uncertainty* (New York: Delacorte Press/Seymour Lawrence, 1981), pp. 4–19, 187–192, 391–418, 427–429.

16. Neal Devitt, "Hospital Birth Versus Home Birth: The Scientific Facts, Past and Present," in David Stewart and Lee Stewart (eds.), *Compulsory Hospitalization: Freedom of Choice in Childbirth?* (Marble Hill, Mo.: NAPSAC Reproductions, 1979), p. 495.

17. Judith Lumley, "Editorial: The Irresistible Rise of Electronic Fetal Monitoring," *Birth* 9 (1982): 150–151.

18. Albert D. Haverkamp et al., "The Evaluation of Continuous Fetal Heart Rate Monitoring in High-risk Pregnancy," *American Journal of Obstetrics and Gynecology* 125 (1976): 310–320.

19. I.M. Kelso et al., "An Assessment of Continuous Fetal Heart Rate Monitoring in Labor: A Randomized Trial," *American Journal of Obstetrics and Gynecology* 131 (1978): 526–532.

20. Raymond R. Neutra et al., "Effect of Fetal Monitoring on Neonatal Death Rates," *New England Journal of Medicine* 299 (1978): 324–326.

21. John C. Hobbins, Roger Freeman, and John T. Queenan, "The Fetal Monitoring Debate," *Obstetrics and Gynecology* 54 (1979): 103–109.

22. C. Wood et al., "A Controlled Trial of Fetal Heart Rate Monitoring in a Low-risk Obstetric Population," *American Journal of Obstetrics and Gynecology* 141 (1981): 527.

23. Jerry Kruse, "Electronic Fetal Monitoring During Labor," *Journal of Family Practice* 15 (1982): 35–42.

24. Mark S. Thompson, Alan B. Cohen, and R. Heather Palmer, "Decision Making on the Clinical Use of Electronic Fetal Monitors," *Seminars in Family Medicine* 3 (1982):89.

25. "Fetal Monitoring: For Better or Worse?" *Harvard Medical School Focus*, December 10, 1981, pp. 1–3,8.

26. Thompson, Cohen, and Palmer, "Decision Making," p. 92.

27. Bursztajn et al., *Medical Choices, Medical Chances*, pp. 20–84.

28. Marilyn T. Erickson, "The Relationship Between Psychological Variables and Specific Complications of Pregnancy, Labor, and Delivery," *Journal of Psychosomatic Research* 20 (1976): 207–210.

29. Bursztajn et al., *Medical Choices, Medical Chances*, pp. 349–388.

30. Ibid., pp. 129–135.

31. Jean Fedrick and N.R. Butler, "Intended Place of Delivery and Perinatal Outcome," *British Medical Journal* 1 (1978): 763–765.

32. Iain Chalmers et al., "Obstetric Practice and Outcome of Pregnancy in Cardiff Residents 1965–73," *British Medical Journal* 1 (1976): 735–738.

33. J.G. Fryer and J.R. Ashford, "Trends in Perinatal and Neonatal Mortality in England and Wales 1960–69." *British Journal of Preventive and Social Medicine* 26 (1972): 1–9.

34. Marjorie Tew, "The Case Against Hospital Deliveries: The Statistical Evidence," in Sheila Kitzinger and John A. Davis (eds.), *The Place of Birth* (New York: Oxford University Press, 1978), pp. 55–65.

35. Sheila Kitzinger, "Women's Experiences of Birth at Home," in Sheila Kitzinger and John A. Davis (eds.), *The Place of Birth* (New York: Oxford University Press, 1978), pp. 135–156.

36. G.J. Kloosterman, "The Dutch System of Home Births," in Sheila Kitzinger and John A. Davis (eds.), *The Place of Birth* (New York: Oxford University Press, 1978), pp. 85–92.

37. W.G. Van Arkel, A.J. Ament, and N. Bell, "The Politics of Home Delivery in The Netherlands," *Birth and the Family Journal* 7 (1980): 102.

38. D. Hoogendoorn, "Correlation Between Perinatal Mortality Figures and Place of Delivery: At Home or in Hospital," *Nederlands Tijdschrift voor Geneeskunde* 122 (1978): 1171–1178.

39. Kloosterman, "The Dutch System of Home Births," pp. 89–90.

40. G.J. Kloosterman, "The Organization of Obstetrics in the Netherlands," *Nederlands Tijdschrift voor Geneeskunde* 122 (1978): 1161–1171.

41. Van Arkel, Ament, and Bell, "Politics of Home Delivery," p. 110.

42. Louise Trusler Mangan and Karen E. May, "Conference Report: Midwifery is . . . A Labour of Love," *Women and Health* 5, no. 2 (Summer 1980): 102–104.

43. Devitt, "Hospital Birth Versus Home Birth," pp. 499–500.

44. Kloosterman, "The Organization of Obstetrics in the Netherlands," pp. 1161–1171.

45. Mangan and May, "Conference Report," p. 103.

46. Ibid., p. 103.

47. Van Arkel, Ament, and Bell, "Politics of Home Delivery," p. 107.

48. Sam Shapiro, Diana Petitti, and Jeanne Guillemin, "The Increase in Cesarean Section Rates: Variations, Risks, and Benefits." Paper presented to the American Public Health Association Meetings, Detroit, Michigan, October 20, 1980, p. 1.

49. J. David Erickson and Tor Bjerkedal, "Fetal and Infant Mortality in Norway and the United States," *Journal of the American Medical Association* 247 (1982): 987–991.

50. Herman A. Hein, "Secrets From Sweden," *Journal of the American Medical Association* 247 (1982): 985–986.

51. Ronald L. Williams and Peter M. Chen, "Identifying the Sources of the Recent Decline in Perinatal Mortality Rates in California," *New England Journal of Medicine* 306 (1982): 207–214.

52. Devitt, "Transition from Home to Hospital Birth," p. 54.

53. Wendy Lazarus et al., *Competition Among Health Practitioners: The Influence of the Medical Profession on the Health Manpower Market*. Vol. II: *The Childbearing Center Case Study* (Washington, D.C.: Federal Trade Commission, 1981), pp. 37–42.

54. Anita B. Bennetts and Ruth Watson Lubic, "The Free-standing Birth Centre," *Lancet* 1 (1982): 378–380.

55. Helen E. Browne and Gertrude Isaacs, "The Frontier Nursing Service: The Primary Care Nurse in the Community Hospital," *American Journal of Obstetrics and Gynecology* 124 (1976): 14–17.

56. Eunice M. Ernst and Karen A. Gordon, "Fifty-Three Years of Home Birth Experience at the Frontier Nursing Service, Kentucky, 1925–1978," in Lee Stewart and David Stewart (eds.), *Compulsory Hospitalization: Freedom of Choice in Childbirth?* (Marble Hill, Mo.: National Association of Parents and Professionals for Safe Alternatives in Childbirth, 1979), vol. 2, pp. 505–516.

57. Margaret Palu et al., "Statistical Outcomes of Elective Home Delivery: II. Comparisons with the Chicago Maternity Center Statistics—Implications for Screening." Paper presented at the International Childbirth Education Association Convention, Seattle, 1976.

58. Mehl, "Outcome of Home Delivery," pp. 93–117.

59. Milton N. Estes, "A Home Obstetric Service With Expert Consultation and Back-Up," *Birth and the Family Journal* 5 (1978): 151–157.

60. Lewis E. Mehl et al., "Evaluation of Outcomes of Non-Nurse Midwives: Matched Comparisons with Physicians," *Women and Health* 5, no. 2 (Summer 1980): 17–29.

61. Erma F. Dingley, "Birthplace and Attendants: Oregon's Alternative Experience, 1977," *Women and Health* 4, no. 3 (Fall 1979): 239–253.

62. American College of Obstetricians and Gynecologists, News Release. Chicago, January 4, 1978.

63. Estes, "Home Obstetric Service," p. 156.

64. Claude A. Burnett III et al., "Home Delivery and Neonatal Mortality in North Carolina," *Journal of the American Medical Association* 244 (1980): 2741–2745.

65. Neutra et al, "Effect of Fetal Monitoring," pp. 324–326.

66. Phillip G. Stubblefield and Jonathan S. Berek, "Perinatal Mortality in Term and Post-term Births," *Obstetrics and Gynecology* 56 (1980): 676–682.

67. G. David Adamson and Douglas J. Gare, "Home or Hospital Births?" *Journal of the American Medical Association* 243 (1980): 1732–1736.

68. Kloosterman, "The Organization of Obstetrics," pp. 1161–1171.

69. Lazarus et al, *Competition Among Health Practitioners*, p. 35.

Appendix 2-A

Detailed Breakdown of Home Birth Outcome Data

Table 2-2 Antepartum Referrals and Transfers

Indication for transfer	Number of patients*	Percent of patients transferred
Breech presentation	14	17.7
Diabetes	5	6.3
Eclampsia	1	1.3
Uterine anomaly with transverse lie	1	1.3
Hydramnios	2	2.5
Placenta previa	2	2.5
Postmaturity	6	7.6
Preeclampsia	8	10.1
Prematurity	8	10.1
Patient more comfortable in hospital	7	8.9
Patient too old for criteria	1	1.3
Patient lived outside hospital catchment area	1	1.3
Weather	1	1.3
Social factors	5	6.3
Fetal demise	2	2.5
Hypertension	4	5.1
Multiple gestation	4	5.1
Thyrotoxicosis	1	1.3
Active genital herpes	1	1.3
Premature rupture of membranes (PROM)	13	16.5
Amnionitis	3	3.8
Urinary tract infection with fever	1	1.3
Total number transferred	79	

*10 patients appear in two categories: 3 PROM and prematurity; 2 PROM and amnionitis; 1 PROM and active genital herpes; 1 postmaturity and preeclampsia; 2 preeclampsia and gestational diabetes; and 1 gestational diabetes and hypertension. One patient appears in three categories: multiple gestation, PROM, and prematurity.

Source: Family Practice Group, Cambridge, Massachusetts, and David Dowis, M.D. and Janet Dowis, M.D., Fresno, California.

Table 2-3 Intrapartum Transfers

Indication for transfer	Number of patients*	Percent of total intrapartum transfers	Percent of labors begun at home
First-stage arrest	23	41.1	3.2
Second-stage arrest	7	12.5	.96
Prolonged latent phase	7	12.5	.96
Prolonged first stage	10	17.9	1.4
Prolonged second stage	2	3.6	.28
Prolonged rupture of membranes	2	3.6	.28
Brow presentation	1	1.8	.14
Amnionitis	1	1.8	.14
Hypertension/preeclampsia	2	3.6	.28
Prolapsed cord	2	3.6	.28
Breech (discovered in labor)	2	3.6	.28
Vaginal hematoma (second stage)	1	1.8	.14
Fetal death (see text)	1	1.8	.14
Total transfers	56		

*Five patients appear in two categories: first-stage arrest and amnionitis; brow presentation and second-stage arrest; prolonged latent phase and first-stage arrest; prolonged rupture of membranes and prolonged latent phase; prolonged rupture of membranes and first-stage arrest.

Source: Family Practice Group, Cambridge, Massachusetts, and David Dowis, M.D., and Janet Dowis, M.D., Fresno, California.

Table 2-4 Postpartum Transfers

Indication for transfer	Number of patients	Percent of home births	Percent of labors begun at home
Maternal			
Retained placental fragment	7	1.0	.96
Atonic uterus	3	.5	.4
Total maternal transfers	10		
Neonatal			
Hyperbilirubinemia	6	.89	.83
Respiratory distress syndrome	2	.3	.28
Fever	5	.8	.69
Cyanosis	1	.15	.14
Polycythemia	1	.15	.14
Imperforate anus	1	.15	.14
Total neonatal transfers	7 (16 indications)		

Source: Family Practice Group, Cambridge, Massachusetts, and David Dowis, M.D. and Janet Dowis, M.D., Fresno, California.

Chapter 3

Midwives and Physicians: Making Home Birth Work Together

Principal Author: Peggy Spindel, R.N.

At the heart of midwifery practice lies the belief that the passage through the birth canal is a healthy experience for both mother and baby. The midwife believes in the ability of a woman's body to move toward health, to compensate for irregularities, and to overcome pain. She sees birth as an expression of spirit in a physical act. She believes that the baby benefits from this creative expression and actually likes being born. For these reasons, the midwife is the practitioner most attuned to the needs of home birth families.

Many physicians—whether because of unconscious fears,[1] training in medical school, or experience in modern obstetrical management—feel differently about the birth process. They look at it from the perspective of disease. They see pitfalls, dangers, disorganization, and disintegration. They believe that birth is violent, something that the baby survives.

There is much of value in modern obstetric science and in the often constructive and sometimes crucial role of physicians in childbirth. Midwives must be thoroughly familiar with advances in obstetric care and must possess many medical skills necessary to recognize and deal with unforeseen complications. When a midwife confronts a problem beyond the scope of her skills, an obstetrician may have the knowledge and responsibility to carry the situation to the best possible conclusion. The backup obstetrician's role is a demanding one, and those willing to take it should be respected and appreciated.

Portions of this chapter have been adapted from George J. Annas, "Childbirth and the Law: How to Work Within Old Laws, Avoid Malpractice, and Influence New Legislation in Maternity Care," in Lee Stewart and David Stewart (eds.), *21st Century Obstetrics Now!* Vol. II (Chapel Hill, N.C.: NAPSAC, 1977), pp. 557–567. Copyright © 1977 by George J. Annas. This version is copyright © 1982 by George J. Annas.

Appreciation is also due those physicians, particularly family practitioners, who pride themselves on providing what comes very close to midwifery care in its sensitivity and point of view. Indeed, they can make excellent home birth attendants, especially in partnership with midwives.

However, midwives and physicians all too often feel threatened by one another, politically and personally. Since medical backup is necessary for home birth, cooperation between physicians and midwives must be recognized as a cornerstone of safe and satisfying maternity care. By understanding the various roles the two kinds of practitioners can (and cannot) create for themselves, it becomes possible to envision the different forms of partnership they can create together.

THE BENEFITS OF PARTNERSHIP

Most birth attendants prefer to work in pairs. Partners need not have identical personalities and attitudes, but they should be comfortable and open with each other. Birth attendants who feel competitive or jealous of each other cannot help but show it to their clients. Each pregnant woman will feel a little closer to one of the attendants, and this preference should be respected and encouraged. Differences in approach to certain situations and differences in personal style bring richness and balance to a practice. In the words of Elizabeth Davis, "True partnership must be defined as a *union* of well-centered individuals, which derives its potency from the blended energies and personal integrity of those involved."[2]

A midwife's hours, extra child care responsibilities, and the legal vulnerability to be discussed in the following chapter may place considerable strain on the midwife's family. In addition, the midwife gives her clients so much caring that her only source of emotional support for herself may be an already overburdened spouse, children, or other close relationships. In organizing her practice, then, a midwife must take many issues and many people into account.

Added to these personal reasons for seeking the moral and logistical support a partner can provide is the fact that doing a birth alone is difficult and risky. It can progress beautifully with a short, uncomplicated labor and delivery, but births cannot be relied on to be short and uncomplicated. Partners can spell each other at a long labor, share in the delivery tasks, talk over what is happening, handle two complications at once, double the support of families, support each other at difficult times, and enjoy the experience together. At moments when difficult decisions and delicate management are required, someone who has been in attendance throughout the labor may be too depleted to respond adequately or, on the other hand, may have a better grasp of the situation than someone who has just arrived. One cannot know in advance which attendant will have the fresh approach, the more accurate assessment, or the critical energy that is needed. Therefore, in planning a home birth practice, a partner is a priority, whether the partner is another midwife or a physician.

Midwives need other midwives to back them up so they can take vacations. Even a small practice is a strain, since a midwife is on call 24 hours a day, 7 days a week. Because the essence of midwifery is a personal commitment to a pregnant woman, vacations need to be planned well in advance. If an overdue woman requires a midwife's services during this vacation time, the decision to attend her or not will be hard. Midwives also sometimes get sick or may have two births in progress at the same time; yet some coverage must be available at all times. Rotating call is a compromise some midwives and families are willing to make.

MIDWIVES IN PARTNERSHIP

When midwives work with other midwives and no physician is present, the belief in birth as a natural, nonmedical event is intensified. The special advantages of midwifery care (such as an empathic prenatal relationship with emphasis on support and education, continuous labor attendance, and a low-intervention approach) are strengthened by midwife teams. Conversely, the positive qualities of medical (physician) care may not be available. These include a broad range of services, nonemergency care of complications, hospital affiliation along with other access to the health care system, and longitudinal care extending beyond childbearing. Therefore, backup relationships assume considerable importance for midwife teams.

Some midwives prefer to work only with other fully qualified primary midwives. This kind of team works well when two complications occur at once or when the clinical situation demands experienced and delicate judgment. However, this arrangement does not give other women who want to learn midwifery an opportunity to do so.

Frequently, therefore, primary midwives work with partners who are not yet fully qualified as midwives but who have the skills necessary to assist. Obstetric nurses can be excellent assistants, as can women who have given birth at home, studied childbirth on their own, taught childbirth classes, and become intimately familiar with labor in the course of providing labor support. Other primary midwives can be consulted by phone when necessary.

The advantages of these two models can be combined by having a third person at a birth. This person should at least be able to identify and set up the various pieces of equipment in the birth kit. In addition to handing the midwives supplies, the third person is present to observe, learn, and sometimes provide labor support.

PHYSICIAN-MIDWIFE PARTNERSHIPS

The physician-midwife relationship in the home birth setting may take several forms. Two of the most common are described here.

The Physician-Nurse Model

The physician-nurse model simply transports the obstetrician-nurse relationship from the hospital to the home. Its main virtue is that it simplifies transfer situations (provided that the physician does not lose hospital privileges or worse, as described in Chapter 4). But the management of birth in the home is complicated logistically and psychologically. First, one would be hard pressed to find a nurse who is used to steady work and steady pay to put up with the irregular hours, low pay, and heavy responsibility of home birth. Second, it becomes increasingly difficult for a nurse, as she grows in her knowledge of normal birth and in her connection with birthing families, to defer to a physician arriving at the end of labor. Third, home birth takes a great deal more time from a physician's routine than hospital birth, even when he or she arrives only at the end of labor. Duties that might be combined with a hospital birth must wait while the physician is attending a birth away from the hospital. The home birth family's need for personal care and a noninterventive approach may be frustrating to a busy, traditional obstetrician. This model seems to work best when it most closely resembles the one discussed below, that is, when the physician is opened-minded and egalitarian; when the nurse is motivated to become a midwife; and when both strive to stay in touch with the needs of the families they care for.

The Physician-Midwife Team

Another alternative, the one used in the authors' practice, is the physician-midwife team. Although the physician takes full legal responsibility, the work is shared, including prenatal care as well as tasks at delivery. The midwife, who has been present throughout labor, can follow through with the delivery with the physician's assistance if the couple desires, or the physician can come early enough to establish the necessary rapport to be primary attendant. Either one can do the newborn examination, although the physician probably will be providing pediatric follow-up. The midwife usually is the one with the time to make postpartum home visits. In the case of a family physician with a practice of which obstetrics is just a part, the physician's time will be more constrained than the midwife's. The physician's role may be shared in a group practice with rotating call. In this case, it is even more imperative that the midwife be available to make a primary commitment to the family. If the physician is a family physician, everyone benefits from long-term contact with the family.

Another advantage of this arrangement is that transfers tend to be less of a shock. Instead of a sudden shift from the home environment to a high-technology delivery setting (sometimes staffed by physicians and nurses with a more interventive outlook), the family will have both the physician and the midwife to advocate for them. A family physician may be able to continue the management of the delivery without calling in an obstetrician. Should an obstetrician be necessary, the family physician can assist (e.g., by scrubbing in for a cesarean or acting as pediatrician for the baby). In supportive settings, the midwife will continue to provide labor support and nursing care. She may even follow through with the delivery if medically possible. It is helpful for the physician to convey his or her respect for the midwife's opinion to the hospital staff.

CONFLICTS BETWEEN MIDWIVES AND PHYSICIANS

Since a midwife is competent to manage normal birth, a physician at the birth is frequently an expensive "extra." If the attendants' opinions differ, the family may feel confused and unsure about whom to listen to. On the other hand, if the two practitioners continue to work as a team, respecting each other's point of view, the quality of care will be improved, not only by providing choices for families but also by achieving a balanced solution that is often better than either opinion.

The midwife gets to know her client as a friend during the pregnancy and sits with her as a sister during her labor. She knows what is happening through her hands and eyes and ears. She can interpret nuances of the woman's behavior because she has been there with her. The physician, either as a home birth attendant or as a backup, has not had this advantage. Some physicians have never sat with a woman in labor from start to finish. Even by attending the labor, the physician will not likely achieve the same intimacy as the midwife unless closely involved in labor support. In this way the "expertise" accumulated by the midwife in a given labor and delivery can lead to conflicts when the physician becomes involved.

A physician may have attended many more births than the midwife, although in a more medical and personally distant way. A medical interpretation of events and aggressive medical solutions to problems may come more naturally to a physician. The midwife's first line of defense when problems arise will tend to be nonmedical means such as positioning, ambulation, or psychological intervention or the least interventive medical option. When, how much, and how long to use either of these divergent approaches is a frequent source of disagreement.

Clients form different types of attachments with and have different expectations of midwives and physicians. The differences may come to light only in retrospect, because couples often do not articulate their expectations. The family may, without being aware of it, put the practitioners in a competitive situation. The father's expectations of the attendant may differ from the mother's. The couple may not even be aware of these dynamics on a conscious level, given people's deep-seated feelings about birth and medicine.

Money can be a bone of contention. A midwife, especially an uncertified one, may make little more than her expenses, while a physician may earn a dramatically greater income (although not generally from home deliveries). Home birth fees themselves are low for midwives (up to $600) compared with those for physicians ($600–$1000). Many midwives are willing to barter their skills and some, in communities such as the Farm in Tennessee, do not receive direct monetary compensation.[3] Unfortunately, only those who charge nothing never have trouble collecting their fees. Physicians have the same difficulties but have more leverage and more often can collect from third-party payers. On the other hand, physicians have higher overhead expenses and more to lose from legal and professional reprisals. Midwives and physicians are also well aware that they are in economic competition.

Authority is another touchy area. Certified nurse-midwives are familiar with the claim that physicians (and only board-certified obstetricians at that) should be in charge of the health care team, including the midwife. How authority is handled in a given relationship will depend on the legal status of the practitioners in the state and the personalities of those involved.

Added to all these possible conflicts are the fundamental differences in temperament, outlook, and perception that can come between any two people trying to work together on a personal level. To cope with these, frank and open discussion is essential, but someone has to take the initiative.

The first hurdle is to convey a feeling of respect for and acceptance of each person on the team. If the physician feels that he or she will never be really accepted by virtue of being a physician, honesty will be hard. A midwife whose skill and judgment are always being questioned will not feel free to share anger or doubts.

Second, protocols for management of common problems such as third-trimester bleeding, prolonged rupture of membranes, or retained placenta, identifying which aspects of management are strict and which are flexible, should be formulated in writing. As less common problems arise, management should be discussed *before* it is instituted by either party, except in an emergency. For example, before sending a woman with mild preeclampsia home on bed rest, a midwife should check with the physician partner or backup about this decision. If the midwife and physician cannot agree, the couple would then have the right to decide for themselves or to seek another opinion, but at least both practitioners would have had a chance to present the pros and cons.

Third, meetings should be held regularly to discuss cases. If the physician and midwife see each other every day at a clinic, they can easily meet once or twice a month over lunch. In a larger practice such as the authors', all the physicians and midwives can meet formally once a month. Apprentice midwives and medical students should be encouraged to join the discussion. Everything is open to review; past and future labors, prenatal care issues, general procedures, particular clients' needs, and conflicts among the attendants and how they can be resolved.

There will certainly be times when issues seem too sharply drawn, when trust and confidence are low and rivalry and conflict dominate. It would be unethical to draw clients into the fray. Others, however, such as childbirth educators, La Leche League leaders, midwife or physician colleagues, or office staff can provide an outlet for frustration and perhaps a channel for communication. A home birth practice without trust is useless to all concerned. It can only function well when trust is reestablished.

CERTIFICATION

Certification is currently available on a national level only for nurse-midwives who have completed training programs accredited by the American College of Nurse-Midwives. There are a few states in which midwifery training other than through the nursing school route can lead to licensure or certification (e.g., Texas, Arizona, and Washington). However, most lay midwives operate without any widely recognized credentials. A very comprehensive state-by-state review of midwifery legislation has been published as a special edition of *Mothering* magazine.[4] (See Appendix B for address for reprint requests.)

The decision to work outside the law is a difficult one. How deeply the midwife must work underground depends on the community. Under these circumstances couples must be carefully screened and the midwife's limitations very clearly spelled out.

The best an "illegal" midwife can hope for is to find (perhaps through a childbirth educator) an obstetrician who respects and supports her and who is willing to take some responsibility for her. This relationship will always be a delicate one, given all the pressures on both sides, and it needs to be nurtured gently.

There are some advantages to certification for lay midwives. A carefully designed program could ensure the public of a *minimum* standard of competence. It could help midwives accept and trust one another. Certification would also strengthen lay midwives' credibility with the medical community.

There are, on the other hand, serious disadvantages to imposing structured control on midwifery practice.[5] A piece of paper cannot provide a client with a guarantee of a midwife's competence. It cannot replace experience, good references, good outcomes, and the high regard of the community. While certification holds out the possibility for responsible control of midwifery practice, it could also serve as a vehicle for overly restrictive or punitive control. Midwifery involves so much flexibility, intuition, controlled risk-taking, and responsiveness to clients' needs that too many strictures could present midwives with the same dilemmas with which physicians worried about malpractice must contend. If certification means medical control of midwifery, most midwives would find it unacceptable.

Recently an alliance between lay midwives and nurse-midwives has been proposed on the national level. Under the tentative title of the Midwives' Alliance of North America (MANA), midwives are discussing common issues such as the definition of a midwife, certification of minimum competency, proposals for training programs, and ideas for fostering cooperation between the two types of midwives. Information about this new organization is available from sources listed in Appendix B.

Where legal certification is unavailable or undesirable, midwives (and their clients) will still benefit from strong *local* alliances. Practice sessions for infrequently used skills can be organized, moral and emotional support shared, and valuable nonmedical second opinions exchanged among trusted peers. High standards of care can be maintained informally by strong local midwives' groups, and those learning midwifery can do so in a positive rather than obstructionist environment.

NOTES

1. Peter Lomas, "An Interpretation of Modern Obstetric Practice," in Sheila Kitzinger and John A. Davis (eds.), *The Place of Birth* (New York: Oxford University Press, 1978), pp. 174–184.

2. Elizabeth Davis, *A Guide to Midwifery: Hearts and Hands* (Santa Fe: John Muir Publications, 1981), p. 24.

3. Ina May Gaskin, *Spiritual Midwifery* (Summertown, Tenn.: The Book Publishing Company, 1978), p. 14.

4. Pacia Sallomi, Angie Pallow-Fleury, and Peggy O'Mara McMahon, "Midwifery and the Law," *Mothering,* Special Edition, 1982.

5. Alan Solares, "Does Midwifery Need Licensing?" *The Practicing Midwife* 1, no. 17 (Fall 1982): 10–16.

Chapter 4

Legal Aspects of Home Birth

George J. Annas, J.D., M.P.H.

The role of the law in childbirth is frequently misunderstood; the law plays many roles, and these roles differ considerably depending on the place of birth. And the law relating to childbirth is changing through legislation, court decisions, opinions of attorneys general, and hospital policy.

The foundations of current law are based on a long tradition of protecting the public against medical quacks and a more recent movement to protect children from abuse by their parents. Since both health care licensure laws and child abuse statutes have ample rationales, independent of childbirth, neither are likely to be abandoned. Those desiring change must thus work for modifications within the framework of these laws. To do this effectively, it is essential to understand the current legal status of home birth.

Since there is very little law directly pertaining to home birth, the conclusions reached in this chapter have been drawn by analogy from a few dozen cases over the past 200 years and from just a handful of state statutes, dealing mostly with midwifery. Nonetheless, three major points regarding the law on childbirth may be made: (1) it is very conservative and is likely to reflect standard medical practice; (2) it is complex and varies from state to state; (3) it is outcome oriented, that is, unless something goes wrong, the law is not likely to be involved.[1]

The state's interest in the outcome of a birth was implicitly affirmed by the United States Supreme Court in the 1973 abortion decisions, which asserted that the state has a strong interest in protecting the life of a viable fetus.[2,3] Thus, while women have a "right to privacy" that prohibits the state from interfering with their use of contraceptives or previability abortions, "the right to privacy has never been interpreted so broadly as to protect a woman's choice of the manner and circumstances in which her baby is to be born."[4]

The standard against which an individual is measured under the law is what a reasonable person would do in similar circumstances. Whether or not it may be considered reasonable in a given case to give (or attend) birth at home is a question of fact. However, it is always considered reasonable to give birth in a hospital, and courts will not force hospitals to change what is accepted as "standard medical procedure" as long as it has the slightest health and safety rationale. In a hospital, a woman's legal control over the birth of her child is almost entirely negative (i.e., the right to refuse all medical interventions, such as anesthesia and episiotomy).[5] She usually cannot demand that the physician practice medicine in a certain way. Although families and consumer groups have been able to influence hospital procedures through cooperative relationships with physicians and through economic competition from out-of-hospital alternatives, legal avenues have not proven a successful route to accomplish change.

Home birth offers the family and the birth attendant greater autonomy at the sacrifice of the legal protection under the umbrella of the hospital. Personnel and procedures not legitimized by the authority of a hospital will be subjected to stricter legal scrutiny in the event of a bad outcome. When a death occurs during a home birth, the district attorney might even decide that a wrong has been committed against society and consider a prosecution for manslaughter. Indeed, except when an issue is made of the unlawful practice of medicine or midwifery, it is unlikely that legal action will be taken against any of the participants in a home birth unless the mother or child dies or is permanently disabled. Also, in the absence of negligence irrespective of site, no criminal or civil action is likely to succeed unless it can be demonstrated that the probability of death or disability would have been significantly lower in the hospital than in the home.

However, the threat of an investigation and possible legal action presents serious issues for those involved in home birth. Physicians, midwives, and families are legally vulnerable in different ways.

A PHYSICIAN'S POTENTIAL LIABILITY

The pregnant woman's physician has a duty to the fetus to provide it (through its mother) with adequate medical care both before and during the delivery. This duty generally does not prevent a physician from participating in a home delivery, but does require the physician to perform standard screening tests to identify high-risk pregnancies, and to take some steps to encourage women so identified to make use of hospital facilities for birth. A physician could be held criminally liable for infant or maternal death in cases of gross negligence or willful and wanton misconduct and civilly liable for malpractice for death or injury if he or she were negligent in the home delivery. However, specific cases are rare.

Malpractice

Physicians' fear of increased malpractice liability for participation in home births is probably based on ignorance of the law of medical malpractice in general, coupled with the climate of fear surrounding home birth that has been created in many states.[6] This ignorance has led to an increase in so-called "defensive medicine," by which physicians allegedly perform certain procedures (e.g., skull x-rays in emergency wards) not because they are medically indicated, but because they think that they may be necessary to disprove negligence to a jury should the patient later decide to sue. A physician taking this "defensive" posture might refuse to do home deliveries on the grounds that hospital births, while unnecessary, are standard medical practice, so that failure to hospitalize might itself be considered negligent. Indeed, at least one physician, a specialist in medical malpractice, has argued in a book on malpractice written for the public that a physician-attended home birth in New York City is itself evidence of physician negligence.[7]

The argument that it is negligence per se when a physician attends a home birth in a community where hospital birth is the standard should be rejected on policy grounds: it does not deter those committed to giving birth at home from doing so but only makes it impossible for them to obtain medical assistance. Legally, a physician attending a birth in the home may, of course, be charged with negligence on any of the same grounds as a physician attending a birth in a hospital. However, so long as the decision to have a home birth is made by a woman after she has been fully informed of the potential risks and complications and so long as all generally accepted precautions have been taken concerning screening and emergency backup facilities, it is highly unlikely that any malpractice action based merely on a physician's having attended a home birth will be successful. In such cases the mother probably will be found to have knowledgeably assumed the risk of home birth and therefore will be barred from suing the physician for offering and participating in that choice.[8]

Indeed, many of the features of home birth described throughout this book make it *less* likely that a physician will be sued for malpractice as a result of a home birth than a hospital birth. There is not only the absence of general anesthesia and invasive medical interventions but also the positive aspects of home birth: individualized care, a well-informed and participating woman, a bond of trust between attendant and family, negotiation of responsibilities, anticipation of outcomes, acknowledgment of risks, mutuality in decision making, admission of errors, and advocacy and support in the hospital if transfer is necessitated. Home birth can be a paradigm case of the process of informed choice that represents both good medicine and the best protection against malpractice suits.[9,10]

Abandonment

A physician will not be found liable for abandonment in a case in which the physician indicates an unwillingness to attend a home birth and later refuses to render assistance when the family calls him during childbirth (as distinct from a situation in which the physician does attend the birth and then refuses to render further assistance). In one case, for example, the physician told a woman requesting a home birth that the only proper place for her delivery was in the hospital, "where proper facilities were available," and refused to attend her at home. She hired a midwife, but complications developed during the delivery and the physician, along with two others, was called. All refused to attend, and the child died. The court refused to hold that the defendant physician was negligent for failing to respond to her call for help.[11]

Administrative and Economic Sanctions

Although physicians are well protected legally, the climate of intimidation that has been created by the medical profession itself in many states is very real. In Massachusetts, for example, the Board of Registration in Medicine considered seriously a regulation prohibiting physicians from participating in home births. The regulation was rejected, not because the board supported home birth but because it did not want to interfere with the way individual physicians desired to practice. The fact that this issue even reached the board is ironic, since at that time (1977) only 200 to 500 home births occurred annually in Massachusetts out of about 70,000 total births—about 7 per 1,000 births, using the highest estimates.

Despite this low incidence, the issue has become highly politicized. The American College of Obstetricians and Gynecologists (ACOG), the American Academy of Pediatrics, and later the American Medical Association adopted official positions against all out-of-hospital births. The past president of the Massachusetts section of ACOG has been quoted as saying that families who have home births are "kooks, the lunatic fringe, people who have emotional problems they're acting out."[12]

Until recently, punitive sanctions by the medical profession against physicians associated with childbirth alternatives fell mainly into two categories. One was the denial of obstetric privileges in the hospital to family practitioners (irrespective of their involvement with home birth); the second was the denial of staff privileges to physicians participating in home births. An example of the second type occurred in November 1976, when the Obstetrics-Gynecology Department of Yale–New Haven Hospital adopted the following "departmental policy:"

> Hereafter (December 1, 1976) any physician with OB Privileges at YNHH who intentionally participates in a non-emergency "home delivery" will be viewed as no longer fulfilling the professional expectations of the OB staff of the hospital, and will immediately have OB admitting privileges revoked.[13]

This policy is legally dubious. It has nothing to do with in-hospital care and, therefore, does not promote the safety of hospital patients. As to nonhospital patients, the hospital has no legitimate concern with their free exercise of the option of home birth. The hospital's interest appears to be economic and may, under antitrust law, represent an attempt to join in a conspiracy to restrain trade (in home births). Finally, the promulgating authority seems ambiguous, and summary revocation of privileges is inconsistent with the "fair administration" policy.

Since 1981 the campaign against physicians who either attend home births or merely serve as backup to in-hospital nurse-midwife services has intensified. Some of these physicians have suffered consequences, such as loss of malpractice insurance; refusal of coverage/backup by other physicians in the area; ostracism by other physicians; loss or suspension of license to practice; wrongful death suits for death occurring during or after home births; and problems with hospital privileges, including refusal of staff privileges. In many cases the physician's participation in home births is not explicitly acknowledged to be the reason for these actions.[14] Many physicians who vocally support childbirth alternatives are under either legal or professional investigation. There seems to be a double standard applied by medical licensing boards, insurance companies, and hospital boards to physicians who support home birth as against those who do not.[15,16]

Criminal Prosecution

When a physician is made vulnerable by a tragic outcome of a home birth, peer pressure may be translated into legal harassment. An example is the case of Dr. Peter S. Rosi, an Alaskan physician who was charged with negligent homicide after a baby he had delivered at home later died in a hospital from meconium aspiration. Four area physicians, only one of whom had questioned Dr. Rosi as to what exactly had happened, notified the state attorney-general and the district prosecuting attorney requesting that he be charged with murder. At the trial, conflicting statistics and testimony were given regarding whether Dr. Rosi had acted properly; that is, whether he had hospitalized the baby soon enough and administered the proper therapy. The physician was acquitted; however, the trial cost him $50,000 as well as damage to his reputation and the threat of revocation of his license. Furthermore, as a result of the pending complaint against Dr. Rosi with the Alaskan Medical Licensing Board, he could not easily move to another state to continue practicing, or move within the state to obtain hospital privileges elsewhere.[17]

A MIDWIFE'S POTENTIAL LIABILITY

When the home birth attendant is a midwife rather than a physician, an additional legal issue arises, that of the attendant's qualifications to attend births. In states that have enacted statutes providing for the licensing of midwives, only those qualifying under the statute can legally practice midwifery. In states that do not license midwives, midwifery is usually governed by the medical licensure statute, and the legality of a midwife's activities depends on whether or not childbirth attendance is encompassed by the statutory definition of the practice of medicine. With this combination of legislative and judicial interest, midwifery law has seen the most activity among the areas of law relating to childbirth.

Unlicensed Midwives

The issue most often raised in midwifery is whether or not it is the practice of medicine, and therefore reserved by law to physicians. In Massachusetts in 1907, Hanna Porn, a trained and experienced nurse and a graduate of the Chicago Midwife Institute, was convicted of practicing medicine unlawfully. The Massachusetts Supreme Judicial Court ruled that "although childbirth is not a disease, but a normal function of women," the practice of medicine is not confined solely to diseases, and obstetrics is commonly recognized as an "important branch of the science of medicine."[18] This conclusion, the court said, was mandated by the state statute on the practice of medicine and bolstered by Hanna Porn's use of drugs and instruments. It would have been different had the state legislature passed a statute that distinguished the practice of midwifery from the practice of medicine.

The next significant case occurred in Texas in 1956. Omar Blake Rowland, who had delivered thousands of babies in the Houston area since 1924, appealed a misdemeanor conviction for unlawful practice of medicine to the Texas Court of Criminal Appeals. Citing the *Porn* case as the only case in point, the court nonetheless found that "the legislature of Texas has not defined the practice of medicine so as to include the act of assisting women in parturition or childbirth."[19] The court found further that a number of other statutes regulating childbirth practices alluded to the role of a midwife as, in effect, a legitimate one. These included a statute authorizing midwives to sign birth certificates. The court reversed the midwife's conviction.

The most recent state supreme court case on this issue was decided in California in 1976. The California Supreme Court held that the legislature had an "interest in regulating the qualifications of those who hold themselves out as childbirth attendants . . . for many women must necessarily rely on those with qualifications which they cannot personally verify." The rationale is that the legislature can reasonably find that the only way to protect the health of the public in the matter of childbirth is to ensure that those who hold themselves out as experts to the public are required to meet certain standards and be licensed. And once the legislature enacts a midwifery statute, anyone practicing outside of its limitations is guilty of a crime (practicing midwifery without a license).[20]

Regulation of Licensed Midwives

The major conclusion from these cases is that the definition of what is or is not the practice of medicine is in the hands of the state legislature, as is the establishment of midwifery as a distinct profession with rules and privileges of its own. Although state laws regulating midwifery vary considerably in their criteria for qualification and restrictions on practice, the dominant trend since the 1970s has been to adopt a statute similar to that in effect in Ohio, which requires that licensed nurse-midwives must hold a diploma from a college for nurse-midwives, pass an examination, be of good moral character, and hold a degree in nursing. Licensed nurse-midwives may work only under the direct supervision of a physician and may not deal with any complicated births, use any instruments, or treat any abnormal condition except in an emergency.[21] The ACOG position is that nurse-midwives should assist only in hospital-based deliveries and that home births should be discouraged. The statutes in a number of states support this position by making it illegal for licensed nurse-midwives to attend home births unless under the supervision of a physician.

Political action has been successful in forestalling rigid regulations in some cases. In 1980 the South Carolina Medical Association (SCMA) drafted legislation that would limit the freedom of midwifery practice by specifying who would be authorized to deliver babies. This was successfully countered by the South Carolina Department of Health and Environmental Control, which approved draft regulations outlining the scope of lay midwifery.[22] In February 1980, the New Jersey Board of Medical Examiners made public a set of restrictive regulations for nurse-midwives which, among other provisions, made it mandatory for anyone choosing a midwife to make two prenatal visits to a physician, restricted midwives to hospital births only, and prohibited midwives from offering services to any woman beyond three months post partum. Owing to strong public opposition, a new set of regulations (issued in August 1980) eliminated the above provisions and made birth centers and births at home acceptable.[23]

Mere passage of a nonrestrictive law does not, of course, ensure professional autonomy for midwives. As De Vries concluded in a study of midwifery legislation, "The receipt of state sanction to practice does *not* bring autonomy, but rather formalizes the dominance of physicians over midwives."[24] State legislatures, while they cannot correct the problem of professional dominance, are the most appropriate arenas for change, and the forum where remedial action is most likely to come in the foreseeable future.

Criminal Prosecution

As with physicians, licensed midwives, operating under the authority of state statute, are held criminally liable only in cases of gross negligence or willful and wanton misconduct, and are held liable only if they fail to perform up to the standards of their profession. Unfortunately, the same unfairness seems to characterize cases brought against midwives as those brought against physicians involved in home births. For example, in 1980 a California midwife was charged with murder as well as with practicing medicine without a license after her first and only mortality in a home birth.[25] And in the same year, after the longest court action in the history of Madera County, California, a midwife was finally exonerated of a murder charge after pathologists testified that the physicians involved were responsible for the death of the baby.[26]

THE FAMILY'S POTENTIAL LIABILITY

People can put themselves at risk with impunity, whether by drinking, smoking, skiing, driving an automobile, or giving birth at home. Generally, there is no legal liability if a mother dies in a medically unattended home birth, since a mentally competent woman is entitled to assume risks to her own life and health. In 1906, for example, the Kentucky Supreme Court decided that no homicide conviction could stand against a husband who failed to summon medical care for his wife in time to save her life during childbirth when the failure was due to his wife's insistence. The wife was well informed and desirous of having her baby at home.[27]

Parents may not, however, take excessive risks with their child's life and health. All states have passed child abuse and child neglect statutes forbidding parents from abusing their children and requiring them to provide their children with necessary medical attention.[28,29] Usually, however, the parents' duty to the child does not begin until after the child is born. There are a few reported cases in 1981 and 1982 in which judges required women to have cesarean sections to save the lives of the near-term fetuses, but these cases are poorly reasoned. Even in the unlikely event that such precedents are followed and near-term fetuses are considered children for the purpose of child abuse and neglect statutes, they would not prevent home birth except in those rare instances when a court order forbidding delivery at home was obtained prior to the birth.[30]

In general, parents may choose the option of home birth with impunity. If, however, they have reason to know that complications are likely to develop that will require hospital care to save the child from death or permanent injury, and if death or injury occurs as a result of the home birth, a zealous prosecutor could conceivably charge the parents with child abuse and possibly with manslaughter if the child dies. The availability of this legal sanction is intended to discourage parents from attempting to manage home births by themselves and to encourage them to seek a licensed attendant at the home birth and to accept hospitalization when it is indicated. If hospitalization or the presence of a physician is reasonably predictable to be necessary to safeguard the life of the newborn owing to a specific prenatal condition or finding, failure to care for the child properly after birth could constitute abuse. In the absence of prior knowledge that complications should have been anticipated, the liability of the mother immediately after birth for failure to take care of the infant is not likely to be great. In at least one case, however, a mother who delivered her illegitimate child alone and unattended in her bathroom was found guilty of infanticide. She failed to tie the umbilical cord, and the baby died shortly after birth from hemorrhaging.[31]

More typically, the father could be held for failure to summon needed medical assistance for the child. In 1905, for example, a Pennsylvania judge instructed the jury that a father could be found liable for manslaughter in the death of his infant for neglecting his duty to summon aid "when the woman was in the pains and perils of childbirth."[32]

CHANGING THE LAW: DEMONSTRATING SAFETY AND REDUCED COSTS

The law is an obstacle to progress in childbirth primarily to those who misunderstand it: Behind both the licensing and child abuse statutes, and at the heart of the home birth and alternative birth debate, are the issues of *health and safety*.[33,34] Since these are legitimate state interests, and since they have special application to children who are otherwise defenseless and could become wards of the state, they (other than ignorance) are the primary issues that must be dealt with to broaden the alternatives available for childbirth.

In the absence of extremely strong public opinion, legislators are likely to widen the scope of a midwifery statute, for example, only if it is shown that the midwives seeking to be licensed can deliver babies as safely as physicians or those midwives already licensed. No other argument is likely to be persuasive. Likewise, in the unlikely event of criminal action against parents for the death of a fetus or newborn in a home birth, the parents can prevail only by persuading the jury that their choice of home birth was "reasonable" in the light of its anticipated safety for the infant.

The law is reflective of currently held medical and societal beliefs regarding safe childbirth practices. The medical profession has succeeded in medicalizing birth to such an extent that some courts now consider it to be "comparable to other serious hospital procedures."[35,36] Most judges and legislators probably still believe that a hospital delivery is less dangerous than a home delivery—even though the opposite may be true with the normal birth. If there is to be a change in the definition of "good medical practice" that courts will accept, alternative birth advocates must either persuade the medical profession to change its practices and recommendations or win enactment of state statutes (or regulations by licensing boards and health regulatory agencies) defining the circumstances under which home or other out-of-hospital births meet the standards of acceptable practice. Such changes in turn will be possible only after enough data can be mustered to demonstrate that the proposed alternatives not only are desired by the public but also are reasonable and safe for the newborn.

In matters affecting the health and safety of the public, the burden of proof is traditionally on those who seek change. This, of course, makes things difficult for the home birth movement, since ample statistics cannot be gathered in many states because of the low incidence of home birth, its unavailability as an option, or the fear of reporting home births due to misunderstanding of the law or local medical society pressures. Nonetheless, the data in Chapter 2 present a case for the safety of home birth, and should provide the impetus for comparative studies on a larger scale.

Congress has indicated an interest in programs that reduce medical costs while improving quality of care.[37] Alternative birth advocates maintain that the alternatives they propose are not only reasonable but also would be both safer and cheaper than standard obstetrical practices. (Supporting data are cited in Chapter 5.) One way to attempt to prove this is through a national demonstration study funded by the Social Security Administration or the National Institutes of Health. It would identify and follow pregnant women and would compare the outcomes for those having home births with the outcomes for a matched sample of women having hospital births as well as those using birth centers. Special provisions should be made to ensure that all participants in the home birth study group have physicians or licensed midwives in attendance if they so desire, that relevant screening tests are conducted and recorded, and that no woman is required to use any setting or birth attendant not of her own choosing as a condition for participating in the project. Only this kind of large-scale demonstration project is likely to generate the quality and quantity of data that will lead to reforms such as the inclusion of midwives among federally-licensed health care practitioners and the inclusion of birth centers and home births as available alternatives under any future national health insurance plan.

Although the trend toward regionalization of maternity care facilities[38] has been viewed as reducing available alternatives and creating economic pressure to bring normal births into high-technology facilities (to underwrite the cost of the complicated, high-risk deliveries performed there), regionalization may instead serve to foster home and other out-of-hospital births. If high-risk births can be screened from low-risk births, and if the facilities for high-risk cases are relatively expensive, there will be considerable economic pressure (at least in a system run by the federal government rather than local obstetricians) to make more economical alternatives available for normal pregnancy, labor, and delivery.

NOTES

1. George J. Annas, "Legal Aspects of Homebirths and Other Childbirth Alternatives," in David Stewart and Lee Stewart (eds.), *Safe Alternatives in Childbirth,* 2nd ed. (Chapel Hill, N.C.: NAPSAC, 1977), pp. 161–181.

2. *Roe v. Wade,* 410 U.S. 113 (1973).

3. *Doe v. Bolton,* 410 U.S. 171 (1973).

4. *Bowland v. Municipal Ct. for Santa Cruz City,* 134 Cal. 630, 638, 18 C.3d 479, 556 P.2d 1081 (1976).

5. George J. Annas, *The Rights of Hospital Patients* (New York: Avon, 1975).

6. George J. Annas, Barbara Katz, and Robert Trakimas, "Medical Malpractice Litigation Under National Health Insurance: Essential or Expendable," *Duke Law Journal* no. 6 (1975): 1335–1373.

7. Richard Gots, *The Truth About Medical Malpractice* (New York: Stein & Day, 1975), p. 48.

8. George J. Annas, Leonard H. Glantz, and Barbara F. Katz, *The Rights of Doctors, Nurses and Allied Health Professionals* (New York: Avon, 1981), pp. 197–198, 251–253.

9. George J. Annas, "Avoiding Malpractice Suits Through the Use of Informed Consent," *Current Problems in Pediatrics* 6 (1976): 1–48.

10. Harold Bursztajn et al., *Medical Choices, Medical Chances: How Patients, Families, and Physicians Can Cope With Uncertainty* (New York: Delacorte Press/Seymour Lawrence, 1981), pp. 349–388.

11. *Vindrine v. Mayes,* 127 So. 2d 809 (Ct. App. La. 1961).

12. Saul Lerner, quoted in Marjorie Harvey, "Homebirths," *Boston Globe Magazine, New England,* Oct. 16, 1977, p. 18.

13. "The Conspiracy of Doctors Against Doctors," *NAPSAC News* 6, no. 1 (Spring 1981): 1.

14. Ibid., p. 2.

15. "Home Birth Physician Cleared in Court, Yet Faces Battle With Licensing Board," *NAPSAC News* 5, no. 3 (Fall 1980): 14.

16. "The Conspiracy of Doctors Against Doctors," p.1.

17. "Alaskan Home Birth Physician Acquitted in Homicide Trial," *NAPSAC News* 5, no. 2 (Summer 1980): 5.

18. *Commonwealth v. Porn,* 196 Mass. 326 (1907).

19. *Banti v. State,* 289 S.W. 2d 244 (Tex. Ct. Crim. App. 1956).

20. *Bowland v. Municipal Ct. for Santa Cruz City,* 134 Cal. 630 (1976).

21. Ohio St. sec. 4731.30–4731.34.

22. "While SC Docs Adopt Stand Against Home Birth . . . SC Bureau of MCH Adopts Guidelines for Lay Midwives," *NAPSAC News* 5, no. 4 (winter 1980): 11.

23. "Public Demand Causes New Jersey Doctors To Back Down in Opposing Midwives," *NAPSAC News* 5, no. 3 (Fall 1980): 23.

24. Raymond Gene De Vries, "Midwifery Legislation: A Case Study of the Relationships Between Legal and Medical Institutions." Doctoral dissertation, Department of Sociology, University of California at Davis, 1981, p. 195.

25. "California Midwife Charged Twice for Same Offense," *NAPSAC News* 5, no. 2 (Summer 1980): 2.

26. "Midwife Exonerated of Murder Charge," *NAPSAC News* 5, no. 4 (Winter 1980): 1.

27. *Westrup v. Commonwealth,* 123 Ky. 95, 93 S.W. 646 (1906).

28. John Robertson, "Involuntary Euthanasia of Defective Newborns: A Legal Analysis," *Stanford Law Review* 27 (1975): 213, 218–230.

29. *State v. Shepherd,* 255 Iowa 1218, 124 N.W. 2d 712 (1963).

30. George J. Annas, "Forced Ceasarean Sections: The Most Unkindest Cut of All," *Hastings Center Report* (June 1982): 22–23.

31. *People v. Chavez,* 1976 p. 2d 92 (Cal. 1947).

32. *Commonwealth v. Signerski,* 14 Pa. Dist. 361 (1905).

33. "Births at Home Create Debate on Safety," *The Nation's Health,* February 1977, p. 12.

34. George J. Annas, "Home Birth: Autonomy vs. Safety," *Hastings Center Report,* August 4, 1978, pp. 19–20.

35. Judge John Paul Stevens in *Fitzgerald v. Porter Memorial Hospital,* 523 F. 2d 716 (7th Cir. 1975).

36. "Note, Family Law—Constitutional Right to Privacy: The Father in the Delivery Room," *North Carolina Law Review* (1976): 1297.

37. Richard Egdahl (ed.), "Quality Assurance in Hospitals: Policy Alternatives." Monograph of Boston University's Program on Public Policy for Quality Health Care, April 1976, p. 4.

38. Committee on Perinatal Health, The National Foundation—March of Dimes, *Toward Improving the Outcome of Pregnancy: Recommendations for the Regional Development of Maternal and Perinatal Health Services* (White Plains, N.Y., 1976).

Part II

Home Birth in Practice

Chapter 5

Home Birth Policy: Criteria for Screening

Principal Authors: Stanley E. Sagov, M.D., and Archie Brodsky

A written statement of policy is a prerequisite for the establishment of a home birth service. The policy statement delineates criteria for eligibility for home birth, conditions under which eligibility is subject to reevaluation, and ground rules to be observed in the attendants' dealings with families as well as with those providing backup services. The policy should be viewed not only as a set of criteria for identifying risk factors that contraindicate home birth but also as a statement of intentions on the part of the attendants. As such, it is a protocol both for clinical screening and for the delicate relationships that must be formed with birthing families as well as with consultants and other supportive personnel and institutions. It is in the context of these relationships that the home birth policy is formulated and modified, and it is on the quality of these relationships that the success of the service largely depends.

UNDERLYING PRINCIPLES

The governing principle of home birth policy is that any circumstance that precludes an unmedicated vaginal delivery, jeopardizes the safety of the mother or baby, or suggests a greater than normal likelihood of intervention rules out home birth. Selection criteria should take into account local and regional variations in the characteristics of the population served (e.g., socioeconomic status, educational level, capacity for informed participation), availability of hospital facilities, ease of transportation, accessibility of consultants, community standards maintained by physicians and midwives, and the degree of institutional and political support for home birth. In the absence of a full-scale support system (such as is outlined in the final section of this chapter), conservative criteria must be employed, by which any complication of the normal course of pregnancy and labor calls for reevaluation of the planned home birth.

A distinction should be recognized between the *statement* of screening criteria in the written policy and their *application* to the individual case. The statement of policy should be worded restrictively, allowing for all possible contraindications, so as to preserve the attendants' prerogatives and to prepare families for the most disappointing eventualities. In practice, however, the criteria may be interpreted with varying degrees of flexibility, as dictated by the data on which the criteria are based, the attendants' clinical experience, and the attendants' personal judgment concerning the woman and family involved. In general, risks can be specified more precisely and judgments made more categorically in the case of observed present complications of pregnancy or labor than in the case of demographic generalizations (e.g., age, parity) or nonrecurrent problems in *prior* pregnancies (e.g., intercurrent illness, breech presentation). Contraindications in the latter categories require finer judgment and allow more leeway for discretion. Nonetheless, the exercise of discretion may be severely constrained by the attendants' vulnerability to professional or legal sanctions in the event of a bad outcome following waiver of their own publicly stated screening criteria. This may be true even when the decision to continue with a planned home birth in the face of an established contraindication has been made with due consideration and (insofar as the probabilities can be assessed at the time) good judgment by both the attendants and the family.

DYNAMIC ASSESSMENT OF RISK

The assessment of risk—and with it of the suitability of the home as the site for birth—is an ongoing one. Beginning in the initial interview, medical history, and physical examination, it continues through the prenatal period, the three stages of labor, and the postpartum course. The criteria used and recommended by the authors for deciding in each of these phases whether the well-being of the mother or baby requires transfer to hospital are summarized in Exhibit 5-1 and discussed in Chapters 7 (Prenatal Care), 11 (Labor and Delivery), and 12 (Immediate Care of the Newborn). In order to be able to exercise responsible clinical judgment, the attendants should reserve the right to cast the deciding vote on the question of transfer. This mechanism for clarifying decision making, especially in the heat of labor, does not take away the family's right and responsibility to articulate its own interests and needs in a collaborative atmosphere.

Although the ongoing reevaluation of the home birth option usually focuses on the possibility of a shift from home to hospital owing to the appearance of unanticipated complications, a change in the opposite direc-

Exhibit 5-1 Eligibility Criteria for Home Birth

I. Contraindications to Planned Home Birth at Initial Screening
  A. Sociodemographic and logistical
    1. Age
      a. Primipara, below 18 or above 35 (see discussion)
      b. Multipara, over 40
    2. Distance from backup hospital too great (over 20 minutes driving time in average traffic)
    3. Physical or emotional inadequacy of home environment as revealed by interviews and/or home visit (see discussion)
    4. Unwillingness or incapacity to undertake prenatal education
  B. Obstetric and medical history
    1. Preexisting chronic diseases (e.g., obesity, diabetes, hypertension, significant cardiac conditions) or emotional disturbances
    2. Grand multiparity (more than five previous births)
    3. Previous cesarean section
    4. Previous birth of a baby with serious congenital anomaly of a probably repeating type that cannot be excluded through antenatal evaluation
    5. Complications in previous pregnancies with an increased risk of recurrence (e.g., documented cephalopelvic disproportion with skeletal contracture)
II. Indications for Antenatal Reassessment of Planned Home Birth
  A. Maternal
    1. Pregnancy-related intensification or unmasking of general medical problems (e.g., gestational diabetes, cardiac disease)
    2. Obvious cephalopelvic disproportion diagnosed by clinical pelvimetry
    3. Preeclampsia (toxemia of pregnancy characterized by high blood pressure, edema, and albuminuria, but without convulsions)
    4. Hydramnios (excessive amount of amniotic fluid) or oligohydramnios (abnormally small amount of amniotic fluid)
    5. Primary or secondary herpes genitalis less than 6 weeks before date of delivery (see discussion)
    6. Inadequate prenatal education requiring reassessment of educational suitability
    7. Psychological instability or social disruption, requiring reassessment of emotional or environmental suitability (see discussion)
  B. Fetoplacental
    1. Uncertain gestational age
    2. Gestation of 42 weeks or more (see discussion)
    3. Multiple pregnancy
    4. Clinically evident cephalopelvic disproportion (e.g., hydrocephalus, macrosomia)
    5. Abnormal placental location (placenta previa)
    6. Abnormal placental function
      a. Intrauterine growth retardation
      b. Evidence of placental malfunction by nonstress tests, stress tests, or estriol levels
    7. Rising anti-Rh titer during pregnancy
    8. Exposure to teratogens (e.g., drugs, radiation, infection, alcohol)

Exhibit 5-1 continued

       9. Persistent breech presentation
     10. Vaginal bleeding of unexplained cause
   C. Maternal or family reassessment of desirability of home birth
III. Indications for Intrapartum Transfer from Home to Hospital
   A. At the time of initiation of labor
      1. Gestation of less than 37 weeks
      2. Premature rupture of membranes (see discussion)
      3. Inaccessibility of hospital for possible transfer (e.g., blizzard or impending natural disaster)
   B. During the course of labor and delivery
      1. Failure of progressive cervical dilatation or descent after trial of diagnostic and therapeutic steps capable of being applied in the home[4]
        a. Prolonged first stage
          1) Prolonged latent phase
          2) Protracted active phase dilatation
          3) First-stage arrest
        b. Prolonged second stage
        c. Second-stage arrest
      2. Passage of dark meconium early in labor
      3. Rising maternal blood pressure
      4. Intrapartum hemorrhage (placenta previa or abruptio placentae)
      5. Fetal distress
      6. Amnionitis (inflammation of amniotic membrane)
      7. Persistent breech or other nonvertex presentation
      8. Persistent abnormal lie (transverse, oblique)
      9. Prolapse of cord
IV. Indications for Postpartum Transfer from Home to Hospital
   A. Maternal
      1. Retained placenta, partial or complete
      2. Deep perineal laceration
      3. Postpartum hemorrhage
   B. Neonatal
      1. Apgar score below 7 at 5 minutes
      2. Apnea or respiratory distress
      3. Anemia
      4. Low birth weight (small for gestational age)
      5. Pathological jaundice (hyperbilirubinemia)
      6. Major congenital anomaly
      7. Metabolic condition
      8. Birth injury

tion may also occur. The family and attendants can reduce risk scores by careful remedial action, as by compensating for prior malnutrition or correcting malpresentations prenatally. A change in the family's preference, either toward or away from the home site, should also be allowed for.

INDICATIONS FOR REASSESSMENT, REFERRAL, OR TRANSFER

The risk factors listed in Exhibit 5-1 are those included in the policy on home births followed in the authors' practice. As a matter of policy, the presence of any one of these factors is regarded as contraindicating home birth, although the decision to transfer in a given case is subject to the discretion of the attendants. Another method of assessing the risk status of a pregnancy is to weight the individual risk factors and calculate a risk factor score according to one of several standard protocols.[1-3]

Discussion of Selected Contraindications

The following issues warrant additional comment, since there is a notable lack of consensus concerning them among home and other out-of-hospital birth services.

Primiparity

Although other home birth services have excluded primiparas, primiparity in and of itself is not a contraindication to home birth in the authors' practice. Families are informed that most intrapartum transfers have involved primiparas, and this fact is considered in the decision-making process.

Home Environment

There are no formal requirements concerning family structure. For example, a woman without a male partner may use a friend or the attending midwife as a labor coach. On the other hand, disruptive unresolved conflict between partners or family members or other evidence of inadequate emotional or logistical support in the family contraindicates home birth.

Herpes Genitalis

Primary or secondary herpes genitalis diagnosed by culture or clinical signs less than 6 weeks before the expected time of delivery is an indication for a cesarean section if the membranes are intact.[5] Such a diagnosis excludes home birth.

Psychological Instability

Current use of major psychotropic medications or a history of institutionalization for psychosis usually contraindicates home birth. In marginal cases (e.g., regular use of minor tranquilizers) a consultation with the woman's therapist may be useful. When neurotic conflicts of some severity are observed, the risks of an emotionally strenuous birth experience at home should be weighed against those of a negative emotional reaction to regimentation and conflicts with authority in the hospital. In some cases a home birth, with its emphasis on self-mastery and affirmation of life, may prove to be a regenerative experience. A home birth may also be viewed as an opportunity for the creation of a therapeutic alliance with the attendant.

Postmaturity

Since function tests (nonstress tests, stress tests, and estriol levels), although useful indicators of the adequacy of the fetoplacental unit,[6] have not been shown to have sufficient predictive value to be a determinant of screening decisions, postmaturity as evidenced by gestation of 42 weeks or more is considered a contraindication to home birth. In such cases, although hospital delivery is planned, the pregnancy continues to be monitored at home with nonstress tests and 24-hour urine estriols every three days. Labor is not induced as long as these antenatal tests are normal.

Premature Rupture of Membranes

Rupture of membranes without evidence of amnionitis or labor for over 24 hours at term poses the same dilemma in home births as it does in hospital deliveries. This dilemma is shared with the family. A traditional approach is to induce labor to avoid the feared risk of infection, which in some instances can be fulminant and even lethal. A less traditional approach supported in some academic centers is to take precautions against introducing infection (no tub baths, intercourse, tampons, or digital vaginal examinations) and to institute monitoring procedures for early detection of infection (oral temperature every four hours and white blood cell counts once or twice daily).

SUPPORT SYSTEMS FOR HOME BIRTHS

The fact that each home birth service must create its own governing policy testifies to the fragmented state of home birth services in America. At the same time, by explicitly acknowledging that home birth is a cooperative activity, such written policies reflect an aspiration to more systematic regional planning for clinical and logistical support. Notwithstanding the enormous political obstacles to the establishment of a maternity care support system in America that gives home birth its due place (obstacles that include not only opposition to home birth but also some home birth attendants' fear of overregulation), it may be a useful exercise to envision what such a system would look like.

An ideal system would recognize the right and responsibility of government and the medical profession to limit the choice of unsafe options in childbirth but not the choice of safe options. It would be built on a foundation of public education, a free flow of information about hospital and out-of-hospital birth among professionals and the public, and free choice within responsible limits. As in most areas of medicine, where there is nothing resembling the polarization that has marked the issue of home birth, data about the various options would be evaluated according to scientific principles, irrespective of the bias of influential practitioners, educators, or institutions. Standards would be maintained (with acceptance of variation within established tolerances) for home and hospital, physicians and midwives alike, with open disclosure of successes and failures and accountability for results. A creative interchange of knowledge and techniques between hospital and out-of-hospital practitioners on an ongoing experimental basis would be encouraged. In this atmosphere, families could make appropriate, informed choices of options in childbirth in consultation with physicians and midwives.[7]

Logistically, the ideal support system would feature an expanded network of home birth support services, both in hospitals and in special mobile units. Backup for home birth would become a matter of established routine in many departments of obstetrics and pediatrics, and hospitals would receive credit on their birth census for home births for which they provided backup (even if transfer were not actually required). Hospital personnel would be made familiar with the home birth option as it existed in their area and trained in the special clinical issues involved in home birth transfers, including those arising from a family's emotional identification with their home as the birth site. Ambulances modeled after the "flying squads" used in Great Britain and other nations would be equipped for cesarean sections and other emergency procedures and would be staffed by experienced personnel trained in emergency decision making, life-support techniques, and nurturance of individuals and families in crisis.

Economic Considerations

The image of ambulances carrying highly specialized personnel and equipment might create an impression of extravagance. Yet in a relatively poor country such as the Republic of South Africa, where one of the authors (SES) was trained, these "flying squads"—fully equipped mobile operating rooms—provide cost-effective, hospitallike interventions, delivered directly to the birth site, for a large rural population. A few ambulances deployed strategically when needed can eliminate the need for many hospital beds now routinely allocated to normal, low-risk births. More generally, out-of-hospital birth promises to reduce health care costs by substituting sophisticated yet voluntary triage for the indiscriminate use of highly trained personnel and costly facilities. Although anyone within reach of a hospital with an obstetric staff can choose this option for a normal labor and delivery, the choice by many families of a midwife-attended or family physician–attended birth outside the hospital should result in savings for these families and for third-party payers and their subscribers. If the safety records of hospital and out-of-hospital birth services are comparable (and Chapter 2 gives preliminary indications that they are), then the economic advantages of the latter must be reckoned with in governmental policy planning.

Such data as there are on comparative costs of existing programs, although far from definitive, predominantly support the projections made here. An English study found home confinement to be more costly than most in-hospital alternatives, but only because it entailed daily home visits by the midwives for a period before and after the birth.[8] A more recent Dutch study concluded that home birth is the most economical form of maternity care in the Netherlands.[9] In the United States, an economic analysis of one home birth in the authors' practice revealed that this birth cost Blue Cross and Blue Shield less than half as much as a hospital birth with a one-day stay and with the same family physician and midwife in attendance and only one-third as much as an obstetrician-attended birth with a three-day hospital stay.[10] (However, the family, which would have been completely covered for the costs of a hospital birth, had to pay the midwife's fee, since Blue Shield reimbursed only for the physician's services in the home.) These findings are in line with those relating to out-of-hospital birth centers. The average cost to Blue Cross/Blue Shield (according to its own fiscal audit) of a delivery in the Childbearing Center of the Maternity Center Association in New York in 1976–1977 was just two thirds of that of an uncomplicated delivery in a New York hospital, while the center's charges were 37.6 percent of those of the hospital and obstetrician.[11] The cost savings that the Maternity Center Association has achieved even as it has compiled an enviable safety record have been confirmed in a report prepared for the Federal Trade Commission.[12] Similar findings have been obtained in a study of 11 freestanding birth centers offering care by certified nurse-midwives with physician and hospital backup[13] (see Chapter 2).

For the economic advantages of out-of-hospital birth to be realized for the benefit of all concerned, there should be unified funding of hospital and out-of-hospital birth services as interdependent units. As a start, birth expenses should be underwritten by third-party and prepaid health insurance plans and government programs without regard to choice of site. A midwife who serves as a primary birth attendant in the home should be paid on the same basis as a physician; a midwife who assists a physician attending a birth in the home should be paid on the same basis as an obstetric nurse. If the health care reimbursement system is to have any rational basis, consumers and providers who save the system money ought to be rewarded, not penalized, for making cost-effective choices.

At the same time, the economic consequences of out-of-hospital birth for hospitals must be recognized and dealt with. A loss of income due to a reduced demand for hospital births would make it more difficult for hospitals to meet the fixed expenses of maintaining obstetric and neonatal services. However, hospitals could made up some of the lost income by providing backup for out-of-hospital births. For this support to be adequately compensated, all of the auxiliary services undertaken by hospitals in a unified birth system (e.g., training programs, standby ambulances) should be taken into account. To defray the costs of keeping personnel, equipment, and space in readiness for infrequent utilization, hospitals should be compensated for all out-of-hospital births under their sponsorship, regardless of whether transfer to hospital takes place. In this way the role of the hospital would not be downgraded but redefined, and the vital importance of the hospital in ensuring the safety of out-of-hospital birth would be acknowledged.

The most prominent statement to date of the need for explicit and systematic allocation of resources in the field of maternity care has been the plan for regionalization proposed by the Committee on Perinatal Health, consisting of representatives of medical institutions and the medical profession.[14] This plan emphasizes medical screening and cost effectiveness to the virtual exclusion of the concerns that have inspired the out-of-hospital birth movement. In contrast, the kind of support system recommended in this chapter has been outlined by Muriel Sugarman,[15] whose alternative plan for regionalization recognizes human as well as medical needs and the variety of ways in which both can be met.

NOTES

1. Arthur J. Rollins et al., "A Homestyle Delivery Program in a University Hospital," *Journal of Family Practice* 9 (1979): 409.

2. Laura E. Edwards et al., "A Simplified Antepartum Risk-Scoring System," *Obstetrics and Gynecology* 54 (1979): 237–240.

3. John J. LaFerla and William F. Rayburn, "Toward a Better Definition of 'High Risk' Pregnancy—The Challenge for Primary Care Physicians," *Seminars in Family Medicine* 3 (1982): 77–82.

4. Emanuel A. Friedman, *Labor: Clinical Evaluation and Management*, 2nd ed. (New York: Appleton-Century-Crofts, 1978), p. 63.

5. Sidney Kibrick, "Herpes Simplex Infection at Term: What To Do With Mother, Newborn, and Nursery Personnel," *Journal of the American Medical Association* 243 (1980): 157–160.

6. Henry Klapholz and Emanuel A. Friedman, "The Incidence of Intrapartum Fetal Distress with Advancing Gestational Age," *American Journal of Obstetrics and Gynecology* 127 (1977): 405–407.

7. Harold Bursztajn et al., *Medical Choices, Medical Chances: How Patients, Families, and Physicians Can Cope With Uncertainty* (New York: Delacorte Press/Seymour Lawrence, 1981), pp. 349–388.

8. John H. Babson, *Disease Costing* (Manchester, England: The University Press, 1973), pp. 44–62.

9. W.G. Van Arkel, A.J. Ament, and N. Bell, "The Politics of Home Delivery in the Netherlands," *Birth and the Family Journal* 7 (1980): 101–112.

10. Mary Lee Ingbar et al., "Choosing Services for Maternity Care and Childbirth: A Case Study" (Worcester, Mass.: University of Massachusetts Medical School, Department of Family and Community Medicine, 1980), pp. III, 50–51.

11. Maternity Center Association, *Childbearing Center: 1976–1977 Cost Analysis* (New York: Health Affairs Research, 1978), p. 9.

12. Wendy Lazarus et al., *Competition Among Health Practitioners: The Influence of the Medical Profession on the Health Manpower Market*. Vol. II: *The Childbearing Center Case Study* (Washington, D.C.: Federal Trade Commission, 1981).

13. Anita B. Bennetts and Ruth Watson Lubic, "The Freestanding Birth Centre," *Lancet* 1 (1982): 378–380.

14. Committee on Perinatal Health, The National Foundation—March of Dimes, *Toward Improving the Outcome of Pregnancy: Recommendations for the Regional Development of Maternal and Perinatal Health Services* (White Plains, N.Y., 1976).

15. Muriel Sugarman, "Toward *Really* Improving the Outcome of Pregnancy: What You Can Do," *Birth and the Family Journal* 6 (1979): 109–118.

Chapter 6

The Primary Care Role

Principal Author: Richard I. Feinbloom, M.D.

Most home birth practitioners will be functioning in the health care system at the primary care level, which is characterized by first contact with the patient (i.e., point of entry into the system); initiation of contact (referral and consultation) with secondary and tertiary levels of care as needed; and longitudinal and continuous participation with the patient regardless of whoever else is involved.[1]

To provide a responsible home birth service the attendant must be sure that a complete set of obstetric services is available. This system should be defined in advance so that consultation and transfer can be achieved smoothly and in a supportive way to the family, attendant, and others involved.

For licensed midwives several kinds of arrangements for this formal liaison may be made. Midwives can form a corporation that hires obstetricians as consultants.[2] A certified nurse-midwife employed by a clinic can use her obstetric staff as backup. A licensed midwife working privately can make a formal connection with a private physician or secure a commitment from the obstetric service of a hospital to provide protocols and rotating backup.

DEVELOPING POLICIES AND PROTOCOLS

Formulating a home birth policy and a set of operating protocols suited to the geographic and professional context in which the attendants must operate requires skill and judgment that is political as well as clinical. It entails the following steps:

- consultation with experienced attendants
- drafting a provisional policy

- modification and approval by support services

The attendants should first seek the advice of midwives or physicians in the same local area (if any) or elsewhere who are experienced in attending home births. These can be found with the help of organizations such as the InterNational Association of Parents and Professionals for Safe Alternatives in Childbirth (NAPSAC), the International Childbirth Education Association (ICEA), and the American College of Home Obstetrics. (Addresses of these organizations are listed in Appendix A.) At the same time, liaison should be established with local childbirth education and alternative birth support groups.

The next step is to enunciate a provisional policy draft and operating protocols based on standard obstetric guidelines as modified by regional and local circumstances and personal judgment. Examples of the screening and management protocols developed by home and other out-of-hospital birth services are readily found in the literature.[3-6] A comparison of these with the authors' guidelines presented in the previous chapter will suggest which criteria represent hard-and-fast clinical consensus and which are more contingent on attitude and circumstance.

To create reasonable working conditions under what may be adverse circumstances, home birth attendants must build alliances by continually demonstrating their skill, responsibility, and good faith to both sympathetic and skeptical colleagues. Toward this end they should present their provisional policy draft to the institutions and personnel whose backup support is sought, that is, the departments of obstetrics and pediatrics at local hospitals. The policy can then be reviewed and modified so as to incorporate the reactions of those whose cooperation is essential.

Collaboration in the development of the policy is only one step in establishing a network of constructive relationships around home birth. The home birth attendants' participation in normal hospital births and in continuing education programs offered by the hospital makes it easier for open-minded physicians and nurses in obstetric and pediatric departments who themselves do not attend home births to serve as allies and advocates. No effort should be spared in removing barriers to productive working arrangements with those who are willing to extend themselves in this way.

Respect and consideration for one's backup consultants (and for the standards of good practice to which they subscribe) are crucial ingredients in making a home birth service work. Moreover, in a climate in which groundless legal or disciplinary actions represent a real threat to the viability of the service, it is wise to assemble a cast of supportive witnesses who will, if needed, testify to the attendants' observance of professional standards.

Following the above guidelines is no guarantee against harassment. Nonetheless, the structure of support that has been built up can be drawn on to cope with harassment and can itself be strengthened by a constructive response to adversity. Attending home births in the United States is of necessity an educational undertaking, and some of the educating is done under stress. Although the stress may involve real threats to the home birth service and to the attendants' livelihood and professional standing, the attendants may also gain an opportunity to clarify issues, to inform the community more widely about home birth, and to strengthen their practice by incorporating the concerns of responsible critics into its protocols.

THE PARTICIPANTS' ROLES

For a home birth system to work effectively, all participants must understand their respective roles. As coordinator of the various functions, the home birth attendant must understand what each of them entails, together with the attendant's own responsibilities toward the individuals and institutions involved.

The Obstetrician

The obstetrician must be available for consultation on prenatal care and especially on the all-important decisions about risk, which will determine the appropriateness of the home as the site for birth. The obstetrician should also be available by phone for questions arising in labor, especially those related to transfer to the hospital.

Families who transfer to the hospital will want to continue to play an active role in decisions regarding their care. The obstetrician should, time permitting, be willing to lay out options, explain the benefits and costs of particular choices, and make recommendations. The obstetrician should be open to the advocacy and interpretive role of the home birth attendant, who may challenge him or her to consider less orthodox alternatives. For example, the attendant may have a more flexible view of the acceptable duration of the second stage of labor, whereas the obstetrician may want to take action when the customary limit of two hours is exceeded.

It is the responsibility of the primary attendant to build a comfortable, trusting relationship with obstetric consultants so as to minimize friction during the management of complicated births. Communication about particular births as well as general issues in obstetrics is an important component of this working relationship, as is acknowledgment of the help provided by one's backup. Clients also should be encouraged to express their gratitude to the consultant when appropriate.

During labor it may be appropriate for the obstetrician and the attendant to confer privately to define the issues and the choices available, and then jointly to present the situation to the couple for their consideration. Differences of opinion or interpretation between obstetrician and attendant can be freely acknowledged. The final decision rests with the family. If the attendant or obstetrician cannot in good conscience support a family's decision, he or she should inform the family of the disagreement, enter a note into the medical record, and, time allowing, seek another opinion.

The Pediatrician

A physician with skills in pediatrics (pediatrician or family practice physician) should be available for consultation by phone and in the home for medical problems of the newborn. This physician can also provide care in the hospital, including the performance of required examinations and completion of required forms. Qualities to look for in such a physician include a low-intervention approach, a positive attitude toward breast-feeding, and willingness to make a home visit.

The Hospital

The hospital must be prepared by the attendants for its backup role. Ideally, the attendants should meet with the nursing supervisor responsible for maternity services. In-service conferences for nursing and medical staffs can be arranged at a later time. The attendants can explain their intention of bringing to the hospital women in labor who have developed problems requiring inpatient care and can acknowledge that such referrals often raise concerns that are related to the hospital personnel's information about and attitudes toward home birth. It is understandable that hospital staff may be upset when they are suddenly confronted by an obstetric emergency that might have been or might appear to have been preventable had the labor occurred entirely in the hospital. Even in the absence of such emergencies the couple that has transferred from home may be disappointed, frustrated, exhausted, and defensive.

The attendants should be prepared to interpret the motivations and values of couples who seek home birth and to provide information both about current research into outcomes of home delivery and about the particulars of the service that they offer (e.g., screening criteria, sharing of risks, prenatal care). At the time of transfer it is the attendants' responsibility to inform the hospital in advance that the family is on the way and, once in the hospital, to relay specific procedural preferences and requests that the family may have.

The attendants must be prepared for a possible overlap in roles with the obstetric nurse. The potential for conflict exists in the absence of prior negotiation. The goal is that the parties view each other as complementary rather than competitive. Specifically, the nurse and attendant should agree to work out a mutually acceptable care plan for each patient at the time of admission.

The attendants should also acknowledge the importance they place on the hospital's support, the appreciation they have for the hospital's availability, and their recognition of the understandable difficulty that hospital personnel may have in enthusiastically accepting the preferences of the assertive minority who choose birth at home. The attendants should make clear that home birth is not tantamount to an indictment of modern obstetrics.

The Anesthesia Service

The anesthesia service of the hospital can be of assistance to the attendant in the selection and use of newborn resuscitation equipment in the home. Ideally this service (or whoever in the hospital is responsible for newborn resuscitation) should be involved in the drills of tracheal intubation with ketamine-anesthetized kittens, as described in Chapter 12.

The attendant should let the anesthesia service know that families are informed about available choices regarding anesthesia, about the constraint that operating room conditions may place on participation of fathers during cesarean sections, and about issues such as the risks of taking oral fluids during labor in relation to vomiting and aspiration associated with the induction of general anesthesia.

The Home Birth Attendant

The previous sections describing the roles of consulting physicians and the hospital have also outlined in essence the primary care function of the home birth attendant. The importance of this role, even when or perhaps especially when other personnel are involved, cannot be overstated. Consider, for example, the case of a woman who requires a cesarean section. Although most home birth attendants will likely perform few or none of the technical aspects of the procedure, the attendant will still be preparing the couple for each step, interpreting what is happening, and providing emotional support. Postoperatively the attendant should visit the woman, communicate observations to the hospital staff and obstetrician, and support the family in its initial adjustment to the baby (including breast-feeding). In discharging this primary care function, the attendant must appreciate the contribution that a knowledgeable, familiar, and trusted individual can make, especially when many others are involved in a woman's care. In these circumstances the home birth attendant is a known quantity in what may seem an alien environment, offering the comfort and reassurance of a relationship that persists even when the surroundings change.

In a case example from the authors' practice, the home birth attendant took 20 minutes in the hospital to prepare a woman who had been transferred during labor to have an intravenous infusion of oxytocin, insertion of a urinary catheter, and placement of an internal fetal monitor with scalp electrode. It was the judgment of the attendant and the obstetric consultants that these measures were necessary if labor were to be safely continued pending evaluation of the need for a cesarean section. The resident in training on the obstetric service, who was inexperienced in family-centered obstetrics, was incredulous and impatient at what he considered an unwarranted delay. In the attendant's view, however, the outcome of the procedures depended at least in part on informed consent, which could be obtained only by careful explanation and a willingness to deal with the emotional concomitants of a traumatic change in plans. It was important that the decision to undertake the interventions indicated be owned by rather than imposed on the woman and her family, so that the sense of guilt and failure that may have accompanied the transfer would not be exacerbated. The attendant sought to help the resident physician understand that it is worth a 20-minute delay to support a family in coping with the disruption of months and perhaps years of planning, as long as the delay does not increase the risk of death or injury to the mother or baby.

Finally, the attendant must be willing to create a climate that promotes regular review of the services offered so that all parties feel comfortable in communicating their positive and negative reactions to the childbirth experience. The feedback obtained is invaluable in clearing up misunderstandings and improving services.

NOTES

1. Joel J. Alpert and Evan Charney, *The Education of Physicians for Primary Care* (Washington, D.C.: U.S. Department of Health, Education, and Welfare, Public Health Service, 1973).

2. Janet L. Epstein, "Setting Up a Viable Home Birth Service Run by C.N.M.'s, Backed by Doctors and Hospitals," in Lee Stewart and David Stewart (eds.), *21st Century Obstetrics Now!* Vol. II (Chapel Hill, N.C.: NAPSAC, 1977), p. 327.

3. Maternity Center Association, *Demonstration Project in Out-of-Hospital Maternity Care* (New York: Maternity Center Association, 1977), pp. 1–4.

4. Lewis E. Mehl et al., "Outcomes of Elective Home Births: A Series of 1,146 Cases," *Journal of Reproductive Medicine* 19 (1977): 281–290.

5. Irene Nielsen, "Nurse-Midwifery in an Alternative Birth Center," *Birth and the Family Journal* 4 (1977): 24–27.

6. Neville Sender, "Changing from Orthodox to Family-Centered Obstetrics," *Journal of Reproductive Medicine* 19 (1977): 295–297.

Chapter 7

Prenatal Care

Principal Author: Richard I. Feinbloom, M.D.

Prenatal care takes on heightened significance in a home birth practice. First, conditions that are harder to deal with at home, such as twins, breech presentation, and maternal diabetes must be detected. Thus, the home birth practitioner has cause for having an even lower threshold for acting on the suspicion of problems than does the hospital-based clinician. Scrupulously attentive prenatal care is the centerpiece of this preventive effort.

Prenatal care also provides an opportunity to promote family well-being in a broad sense. Educational concerns (extending beyond pregnancy and birth) and an emphasis on self-care are part of the prenatal relationship with the home birth attendant as well as of the childbirth education classes, which are discussed in Chapter 8. Another goal of prenatal care is the cultivation of the trust needed for informed choice and shared decision making.

The relationship between the couple and the attendants is collaborative, each having unique attitudes and knowledge to share with the other in working toward a common goal.[1] The prospective mother and father have individual sensitivities, strengths, and weaknesses, knowledge of which is as useful for the attendants as are measurements of blood pressure and uterine size. In turn, the attendants share their technical knowledge and experience gained in working with other families. It takes time to get to know each other, and in a physician-midwife practice the midwives tend to be the ones who invest this time, which amounts to 6 to 12 hours prior to delivery.

INITIAL VISITS

The family and attendants begin preparations for a home birth by exchanging the information necessary to establish ground rules for a collaborative relationship. Having established a contract to work together, they proceed with an intake assessment (complete history, laboratory tests, physical examination) and oral and written briefings about the prenatal course.

Information and Agreements

The purpose of the initial meetings is to determine whether there is sufficient congruence of interests for the parties to come to an agreement to work together. At this time the prospective clients' needs are explored and the attendants' services are explained. The meeting is an opportunity for the parties to begin to get to know each other and clarify their values and intentions. The attendants must articulate their policy and practice on a number of crucial issues, so that the family will know what to expect and how they should prepare themselves to participate. Some of these questions require agreement on principle as well as procedure.

- *characteristics of the attendants.* What are the roles of the physicians and/or midwives in the practice? Can the family choose a primary attendant?
- *prenatal visits.* What is the schedule of prenatal visits? Are family members encouraged to be present?
- *childbirth education.* What opportunities and requirements are there concerning attendance at childbirth classes? (See Chapter 8.)
- *analgesia.* Are analgesic medications brought to the home? Under what circumstances are they used?
- *technical procedures.* What procedures are performed routinely? What emergency equipment is brought to the home?
- *decision-making authority.* In the event of a disagreement between the family and the attendant, who casts the deciding vote?
- *transfer to hospital.* Under what circumstances is transfer to hospital likely to be initiated? How is it managed? What are the responsibilities of all parties?

Discussion of Risk

The choice of a home or hospital birth is a choice between risks in a world where uncertainty is inherent in all decisions and activities.[2] To provide an appropriate context for this choice on the part of the family, the attendant should summarize the information presented in Chapter 2 on the risks of home and hospital birth. These risks—and in particular the consequences of the minority choice of home birth—are shared by the family and the attendants. By raising at the outset this issue of shared responsibility, the attendants can acknowledge and delimit their own responsibility while helping the family acknowledge and cope with theirs.

Materials and Instructions

If the family and attendants are able to reach the working agreements necessary for a home birth, a medical record is initiated. The family is given the following materials:

- policy statement on home birth (see Chapter 5)
- schedule of prenatal visits (see example included in this chapter)
- dietary plans
- comprehensive health questionnaire for the woman
- family history form for both partners
- list of required supplies (see Chapter 10)
- booklet on fetal growth and development
- release forms for past medical records
- fee schedule

At this time the woman is offered a prescription for prenatal vitamins or for iron (60 to 100 mg elemental iron per day supplied either as ferrous sulfate 300 mg, ferrous fumarate 200 mg, or ferrous gluconate 435 mg, once or twice daily) and folate (folic acid 1.0 mg once daily). She is asked to keep a three-day written record of her diet, which is reviewed at the next visit when the question of optimal weight gain in pregnancy is also discussed. These dietary issues are treated in greater detail in later sections of this chapter.

The History

Together with the physical examination and laboratory studies, the history is part of an intake assessment to which one hour is normally allotted. The history may be taken during the initial visit or the following one.

General Medical History

The woman's medical history is reviewed. The review can begin with broad questions, such as "Have you ever had any major medical problems?'' ''Have you ever been hospitalized, and, if so, for what?'' ''Have you had any operations?'' ''Are you taking any medications on a regular basis?'' ''Do you use alcohol or any other drug taken for pleasure?'' ''How would you judge your overall health to be?'' ''Are you under care for any problem now by a physician, chiropractor, therapist, or healer of any kind?''

The answers to these broad questions are supplemented by the answers given to the medical history questionnaire and more focused questions relating to specific organ systems listed on the prenatal history form. Information obtained from previous medical records is integrated into the history. Positive responses are assessed in terms of how the identified problem might affect the pregnancy and vice versa.

Reproductive History

The obstetrical history reviews and characterizes each past pregnancy including the following:

- year of occurrence
- problems during pregnancy
- outcome (live birth, abortion, stillbirth)
- use of anesthesia or other medication
- episiotomy
- electronic fetal monitor
- intravenous infusion
- type of delivery (vaginal, cesarean section)
- complications of labor and delivery
- gestational age and weight of newborn
- condition of infant at birth and in the perinatal period
- maternal problems in the postpartum period
- current condition of child if living

Also solicited and noted are the couple's perceptions of the quality of the birth and of their interactions with attendants and (if applicable) hospital staff. Information from past medical records is integrated into the obstetric history.

A couple is considered to be at increased risk of either one or both partners having a chromosomal abnormality (usually a translocation) if they have had either three or more consecutive spontaneous first-trimester fetal losses or one or more spontaneous first-trimester fetal losses plus a stillborn or liveborn child with a congenital malformation. Such a couple are considered candidates for chromosomal analyses. If these are abnormal, the present and subsequent fetuses should have chromosomal analyses because of the increased risk (in the case of gestations which go to term) of having an affected baby.

The menstrual history includes menarche, regularity of cycles, intervals between cycles, and length of cycles. Traditionally, the estimated date of "confinement" (in a lying-in hospital) is calculated from the last menstrual period on the assumption of an average 28- to 30-day cycle. For longer or shorter cycles, more accurate dating uses the estimated date of ovulation, which is considered to be 14 days prior to the next expected period. Many women are very attuned to their ovulations, making this biologic event a reliable marker for conception.

Dating the pregnancy as accurately as possible takes on added importance in a home birth, since both prematurity and postmaturity pose problems that are harder to deal with at home. Besides the last menstrual period, other useful markers of the age of gestation are the quickening (the woman's perception of fetal movement) at about 18 to 20 weeks in a primigravida and 16 to 18 weeks in a multigravida, the first hearing of the fetal heart tones with a fetoscope at about 16 to 20 weeks, and the measured size of the uterus. Any uncertainty about or discrepancies in the above indicators of the time of gestation can be resolved by discriminating use of ultrasound. The ease or difficulty of conception is noted. For example, a history of infertility and many years of "trying" might predict a heightened level of anxiety, which may affect the subsequent course of the pregnancy.

Family History

A family history is obtained, starting with any children of the couple and working back along a branching family tree to their grandparents. Each family member is identified by date of birth, major medical problems, and age at and cause of death. Stillbirths should be included. Particular attention is paid to congenital anomalies, mental retardation, proven chromosomal aberrations, and other diseases that have a hereditary basis. Additional information on family members both living and dead may be obtained through old medical records. The risk of recurrence of an abnormality present in a previous child of the couple (e.g., clubfoot or cleft palate) can be estimated, even though in many instances prenatal detection by present techniques is not possible. A genetics consultation should be obtained early in the pregnancy when there is any question of a genetically transmitted disorder. A good general reference on genetic problems for both the attendant and family is *Know Your Genes* by Aubrey Milunsky.[3]

A family history of multiple births should also be noted because of the tendency of this pattern to repeat and the desirability of avoiding such births at home because of increased fetal and maternal risk.

The racial and ethnic identity of the partners is also important in identifying individuals at higher risk of carrying recessive traits, those which can become manifest only through the mating of two carriers. Two relatively common recessive disorders for which parental carriers can be identified and the affected fetus detected in utero are Tay-Sachs disease in Jews of Ashkenazi (eastern European) origin and sickle cell anemia in blacks.

Increasing maternal age predicts increased risk of Down's syndrome (mongolism). At age 20 the risk is 1 per 2,000; at 30, 1 per 1,000; at 35, 1 per 365; at 40, 1 per 100; at 45, 3 per 100. A positive family history of this disorder, which suggests the rarer hereditary form of Down's syndrome, should prompt a chromosomal analysis first of the affected relative and then (if this is positive for a translocation of chromosomes) of the woman and her partner for the carrier state. The standard recommendation is to perform an amniocentesis at 14 to (preferably) 16 weeks of gestation on women who are aged 35 and above or are known carriers of Down's syndrome in order to detect this chromosomal disorder in utero. The decision to undergo testing is the couple's and must include consideration of the risk of inducing abortion through amniocentesis (about 0.5 percent in the best hands).[4] Information needed for informed choice should be made available early in the pregnancy.[5]

Another genetic disorder that can affect the well-being of the fetus (and that may also affect future pregnancies) is that of discrepant Rh blood types, in the case in which the mother is Rh negative and the father is Rh positive. Rh testing of the mother and, at times, of the father is part of prenatal laboratory testing.

The family history is also important in identifying the woman at increased risk of gestational diabetes. The presence of diabetes in parents, siblings, aunts, or uncles is considered significant.

Laboratory Studies

The routine laboratory studies recommended for all pregnant women include the hematocrit; blood type, Rh determination, and irregular antibody screen;[6] rubella antibody titer; urine test for protein and glucose; urine culture;[7-9] serological test for syphilis; and the Papanicolaou smear of the uterine cervix. Other tests commonly performed are determination of maternal alpha-fetoprotein,[10] culture of the uterine cervix for gonococci, and serological testing for toxoplasmosis.[11] Detailed discussions of these tests and their use in pregnancy can be found in standard texts. Since the implications of the tests for the management of pregnancy and labor are subject to change, protocols should be developed with consultants.

Physical Examination

The physical examination provides the attendant with essential information and offers an important educational opportunity for the woman and her partner. Useful adjuncts to the examination are anatomical drawings, a model of the pelvis, and a hand mirror. The examination also represents the first physical contact between attendant and woman. This "laying on of hands" is an important ingredient in providing care.

A complete general and pelvic examination is performed, including visualization of the optic fundi and the testing of deep tendon reflexes. The examiner can enhance the value of the examination for the couple by describing each step and its rationale. Women and their partners greatly appreciate a running commentary on what is done, why it is done, and what is found. Inquiry can be made about health practices such as breast examination and flossing of teeth as the relevant parts of the body are examined.

In the authors' practice, stirrups are not routinely used for the pelvic examination. Instead, the supine woman places her feet at the corners of the examination table and moves her buttocks as close to the edge as comfort will allow. The woman and her partner are encouraged to visualize the vagina and cervix with the speculum and hand mirror.

The results of the examination are shared with the couple and recorded on the physical examination form. After the completion of the history, basic laboratory work, and physical examination, a risk assessment is made according to one of the protocols referenced in Chapter 5. The risk assessment is shared with the woman and her partner. Only pregnancies categorized as low risk are considered suitable for home delivery.

Problem and Medication Lists

Following completion of the intake assessment, a problem list is constructed using the problem-oriented medical record system. This system helps the attendants organize information and avoid errors of omission. The list is updated as the problems change.

All medications including prenatal vitamins are entered by date on a separate medication sheet. The medications are numbered to correspond to the problems on the problem list.

Prenatal Briefings

During the initial visits, information is provided concerning preventive measures and other aspects of self-care during pregnancy. Areas covered include teratogens, automobile safety, physical fitness, and sexual activity.

Teratogens

Drugs and Medications. *All* drugs are considered to be potential teratogens. The woman is encouraged to check with the attendant before using any drug, over-the-counter or otherwise. The reader is referred to standard sources for lists of common drugs that might be needed in pregnancy and the risks of each.[12]

Alcohol. Alcohol is a teratogenic drug especially in high doses and when acting in combination with other drugs. Although moderate drinking has not conclusively been demonstrated to cause birth defects,[13] the best recommendation is to avoid ingestion of alcohol during pregnancy, *especially during the first trimester,* pending further study.

Tobacco. Cigarette smoke constitutes a significant risk to the fetus in utero.[14–18] Pregnant women who smoke are strongly urged to stop because of the toxic effects of cigarette smoke both before and after birth, as well as the fact that the parents will soon be role models for the child.

X-rays. Prospective parents can be reassured that there is no good evidence that x-rays, in the doses used in diagnostic radiology, are teratogenic. Nonetheless, unnecessary x-rays are avoided during pregnancy. Necessary radiography is performed with the uterus shielded.

Pets. Parents are briefed on issues such as the risk of toxoplasmosis from cat litter and the precautions to be taken.

Automobile Safety

The importance of seatbelt use in automobiles is stressed. In this country automobile accidents constitute a major risk in morbidity and mortality to women of childbearing age. During pregnancy, automobile-related injuries are a major threat to both mother and fetus. As far as possible, the shoulder harness and lap belt should be positioned above and below the uterus respectively. All passengers need to be restrained, not just the pregnant woman. A crash will send unbelted passengers flying within the car, risking injury to themselves and others.

Guidance on the selection and use of crash-tested, properly installed infant and child restraints is also offered. For this purpose the booklet

"Don't Risk Your Child's Life" has been found to be useful to families (see Appendix B).

Exercise and Sexual Activity

During the initial visits the woman and her partner are informed about the prenatal exercises described in detail in Chapter 9, with emphasis on the perineal muscle-strengthening Kegel maneuver. It is pointed out that Kegel exercises are part of the tradition of female hygiene in many non-Western cultures, passed on from mothers to daughters.

Regarding sexual activities, the couple is encouraged to do what is comfortable for them. There are no specific prohibitions against coitus. Although one study has shown that intercourse during the last weeks of pregnancy was associated with increased intrauterine infections,[19] a definitive answer to this question is not available. Pregnant women and their partners should be informed of the controversy over this issue.

Pregnancy is also a time to acknowledge that lovemaking is not to be equated with sexual intercourse. The couple is encouraged to explore noncoital ways of expressing sexual feelings (with respect, of course, for their cultural and religious values). Suggested readings for couples are provided in Appendix C.

Checklist for Initial Prenatal Visits

The protocols given in this section for initial visits are summarized in Exhibit 7-1.

SUBSEQUENT PRENATAL VISITS

Following the initial examination, prenatal checkups typically are scheduled every 4 weeks until 32 weeks, at 34 and 36 weeks, and weekly thereafter until delivery. On each visit, an interval history is taken. This history might begin with an open-ended question addressed to both partners, such as "How are things going?" The attendant can also inquire about the perceived well-being of the baby by asking, "And how has the baby been?" Such an inquiry acknowledges the baby to be an active, increasingly important participant in the family. Inquiry can also be made into dreams and fears about the baby or the pregnancy, worries about acts of commission or omission that might affect the fetus, and good feelings that arise. It is also valuable to provide an opportunity for the couple to express any concerns that have not already been addressed: "Were there any other questions you wanted to bring up?"

Exhibit 7-1 Checklist for Initial Prenatal Visits

---

1. Discussion of risks, expectations, and responsibilities of the woman and her partner
2. Complete history and physical examination including pelvic assessment
3. Review of general medical questionnaire
4. Review of family history tree of both partners
5. Papanicolaou test
6. Gonorrhea culture
7. Complete blood cell count
8. ABO and Rh blood typing, Rh antibody titer, determination of irregular antibodies
9. Serological test for syphilis
10. Rubella titer
11. Initiation of prenatal forms for hospital to allow for smooth transfer if necessary
12. Initiation of a three-day dietary history and provision of nutritional guidelines
13. Initiation of contact with midwife
14. Prescription for prenatal vitamins or iron and folate
15. Discussion of teratogens (e.g., medications, alcohol, tobacco), auto safety, and physical fitness
16. Instruction in self-care (e.g., dental hygiene)
17. Genetic screening tests as indicated (e.g., sickle cell anemia, Tay-Sachs disease)
18. Urine culture, protein, glucose.

At each visit the woman is weighed, her urine is checked for protein and glucose, and her blood pressure is taken. Once the uterus has risen out of the pelvis, its size is measured; the presentation, lie, and position of the baby are determined; the point of maximum intensity of the fetal heart tones is located; and the presence or absence of edema is noted.

It is helpful to carry on a running commentary about what the attendant is doing and why. Examination findings, such as feeling the head, are described, and the couple is encouraged to check these for themselves. When unsure about a finding, the attendant should ask a colleague in the office to check it also, thus demonstrating the value of a second opinion.

Some women enjoy weighing themselves and checking their own urine. Some also like to keep records for their own use. Such participation is to be encouraged.

Weight Gain

The goal for weight gain in pregnancy is between 25 and 35 pounds. A gain of less than 15 pounds by 36 weeks is considered cause for concern. It correlates with fetal growth retardation, places the pregnancy in a high-risk status, and probably should disqualify the home as a site for delivery. A gain of greater than 1 pound per week after 36 weeks has been regarded traditionally as predictive of preeclampsia and has prompted initiation of preventive measures. A gain of 2 or more pounds in 1 week or 6 or more pounds a month, particularly between the 20th and 30th weeks of gestation, has been considered by many authorities to be indicative of preeclampsia.

Recently the significance of weight gain in predicting fetal mortality and morbidity (whether or not related to preeclampsia) has been called into question. In a review of 38,636 pregnancies and births, one group of investigators found that in the third trimester neither maternal weight gain (except for lack of weight gain) nor edema alone was predictive of increased fetal mortality.[20,21] This interpretation has been challenged by another analysis of the same study population that found that women who were overweight at the start of pregnancy had the fewest fetal and neonatal deaths when they had a 16-pound maximum weight gain at term. Optimal weight gain for "normal" mothers was 20 pounds and for "underweight" mothers was 30 pounds.[22]

In the authors' judgment, precise guidelines for defining pathological weight gain during pregnancy are still not available. Although the commonly recommended upper limit is 35 pounds, many women gain more without adverse consequences. Nonetheless, weight gains of greater than 35 pounds are likely to result in larger babies, with increased risk of cephalopelvic disproportion and its attendant consequences, including a higher rate of cesarean sections. Another result of excess weight gain is increased risk of gestational diabetes, as detailed in the following section. In the authors' practice, an increase in weight of more than 2 pounds per week, even as an isolated finding, alerts us to the possibility of pathological fluid retention, increases our monitoring for signs of preeclampsia, may lead us to initiate measures to prevent preeclampsia, and is taken into account in determining the advisability of home birth.

How strenuous an effort should be made to limit weight gain to the guidelines described is not clear at present. The authors' position is that a woman should eat what she needs of a well-balanced diet to satisfy her appetite but should not allow herself to become obese. If she is obese at the onset of pregnancy, she should be encouraged to avoid further increases in obesity by correcting poor eating and exercise habits but should not put herself on a reducing diet. Women who are considered to be at increased risk for gestational diabetes by the criterion of weight need careful nutritional counseling to limit weight gain in pregnancy.

Nutritional Evaluation and Counseling

It is essential that the attendant be familiar with the basic physiology of eating, some elementary chemistry of digestion, the various nutrients and their uses, daily requirements for pregnancy and lactation, the four food groups, cooking and meal planning, and identification of nutritionally high-risk women.

There are many methods available to screen for dietary inadequacy in pregnancy and to intervene to improve maternal nutrition. They are usually based on a three day log of the diet or, less desirably, a history taken from 24-hour recall. The history should include type and quantity of food and liquids, method of preparation, and time of day when eaten. Specific inquiry is made concerning medications (prescribed and over-the-counter), vitamins, alcohol, cigarettes, or illicit drugs. Information on the mother's exercise and work schedule, prepregnancy weight, hematocrit or hemoglobin, and obstetric condition should be taken into consideration. The diet may be evaluated by nutrients or by servings of food groups. In communicating the evaluation to the woman, the strengths of her diet should be emphasized while its weaknesses are tactfully pointed out.

The "Higgins Intervention Method for Nutritional Rehabilitation During Pregnancy"[23] is frequently used by nurse-midwives and is excellent for nutritionally high-risk populations. The California Department of Health Services offers an excellent booklet on nutritional assessment and intervention, which includes tables, charts, and clinical forms, such as Tables 7-1 and 7-2 and Exhibit 7-2 (see Appendix B). An advantage of this booklet is its adaptation of nutritional requirements to different cultures. Also useful is an authoritative reference such as the *Handbook of the Nutritional Contents of Foods*,[24] prepared for the U.S. Department of Agriculture. It includes almost 2,500 foods. Many books written for the general reader give excellent information on nutritional contents of foods, protein complementarity, vegetarian or macrobiotic diets and pregnancy, recipes, meal planning, and maintaining good nutrition on a budget (see Appendix C).

A booklet that is inexpensive enough to give to all clients at their initial prenatal visit is *As You Eat So Your Baby Grows: A Guide to Nutrition in Pregnancy* by Nikki Goldbeck,[25] which includes practical information for pregnant women, such as a chart on protein complementarity and lists of foods containing essential nutrients.

Many women find the recommended allowances for pregnancy too much to consume. The attendant should help these women choose foods with a higher nutritional concentration. Women with nausea and vomiting or other gastrointestinal discomforts need special counseling. An attendant should find a nutritionist to assist in difficult cases if required.

One should be flexible on the issue of vitamins and other supplements as long as nutritional requirements are being met. Some women buy supplements either in combination or separately, while others refuse supplements altogether.

Table 7-1 Recommended Daily Dietary Allowances for Pregnancy[1]

	Age			
	11–14	15–18	19–22	23–50
Body size				
Weight kg	44	54	58	58
lb	97	119	128	128
Height cm	155	162	162	162
in	62	65	65	65
Nutrients				
Energy, kcal	2700	2400	2400	2300
Protein, gm	74	78	76	76
Vitamin A, RE[2]	1000	1000	1000	1000
IU[2]	5000	5000	5000	5000
Vitamin D, IU	400	400	400	400
Vitamin E, activity, IU	15	15	15	15
Ascorbic Acid, mg	60	60	60	60
Folacin, µg	800	800	800	800
Niacin, mg[3]	18	16	16	15
Riboflavin, mg	1.6	1.7	1.7	1.5
Thiamin, mg	1.5	1.4	1.4	1.3
Vitamin B$_6$, mg	2.5	2.5	2.5	2.5
Vitamin B$_{12}$, µg	4.0	4.0	4.0	4.0
Calcium, mg	1200	1200	1200	1200
Phosphorus, mg	1200	1200	1200	1200
Iodine, µg	125	125	125	125
Iron, mg[4]	18+	18+	18+	18+
Magnesium, mg	450	450	450	450
Zinc, mg	20	20	20	20

[1] Adopted from Food and Nutrition Board, National Research Council, National Academy of Sciences, *Recommended Dietary Allowances*, Eighth Edition, Washington, D.C., 1974.

[2] RE = Retinal Equivalent; IU = International Unit. The recommended unit of measure is RE. 1 RE = 10 IU.

[3] Although allowances are expressed as niacin, it is recognized that on the average 1mg of niacin is derived from each 60mg of dietary tryptophan.

[4] This increased requirement for pregnancy cannot be met by ordinary diets; therefore, the use of supplemental iron is recommended.

Source: Reprinted from *Nutrition During Pregnancy and Lactation*, with permission of the California Department of Health Services, © 1975.

Table 7-2 Daily Food Guide

	Number of servings		
Food group	Nonpregnant woman	Pregnant woman	Lactating woman
Protein foods			
Animal*	2	2	2
Vegetable†	2	2	2
Milk and milk products	2	4	5
Breads and cereals	4	4	4
Vitamin C–rich fruits			
and vegetables	1	1	1
Dark green vegetables	1	1	1
Other fruits and vegetables	1	1	1

*1 serving is 2 oz. (60 g).
†Should include at least 1 serving of legumes.

Source: Reprinted from *Nutrition During Pregnancy and Lactation* with permission of the California Department of Health Services, © 1977.

Exhibit 7-2 Nutritional Risk Factors in Pregnancy

Adolescence
High parity
Frequent conceptions
Low prepregnancy weight
Insufficient weight gain during pregnancy
Obesity
Previous obstetric complications
Existing medical complications
Dietary faddism and pica
Low income
Ethnic and/or language differences
Excessive smoking, alcoholism, and drug addiction
Psychological conditions

Source: Reprinted from *Nutrition During Pregnancy and Lactation* with permission of the California Department of Health Services, © 1975.

Urine Test for Protein and Glucose

The urinary protein and glucose may be determined by Uristix (Ames) dipstick.

Proteinuria

A protein reading of negative, trace, or 1 + in pregnancy is generally accepted as normal; 2 + or greater is considered abnormal. Also significant is a shift of two or more levels: from negative to 1 +, from trace to 2 +, 1+ to 3 +, or 2+ to 4 +.[26] With abnormal degrees of proteinuria by "dipstick," some authorities suggest performing a quantitative determination.[27] The presence of at least 300 mg protein in a 24-hour urine collection or a midstream voiding of 1 gm or more protein per liter of urine on two or more occasions at least six hours apart is considered significant.

In determining the significance of proteinuria, so-called "benign" or "postural" proteinuria must be excluded. Benign (postural) proteinuria is believed to be due to impingement of the gravid uterus on the renal veins and should clear when urine is collected with the woman in a lateral recumbent position. The finding of nonpostural proteinuria of 2 + or more is considered significant and is regarded as a factor arguing against a home birth.

Urine Glucose: Screening for Gestational Diabetes

The urine glucose test is used to identify women at risk for gestational diabetes. There is some difference of opinion about when to regard glycosuria as significant. It has been pointed out that glycosuria is common in normal pregnancy, resulting as it does from increased glomerular filtration and decreased resorption of glucose. Seventy percent of women may demonstrate glycosuria at some time, while only 17 percent will have two positive urine samples, and only 1 percent will have an abnormal glucose tolerance test.[28] Therefore, it has been suggested by some clinicians that only those women with two or more separate urine tests positive for glucose be evaluated with an oral glucose loading test.

Gestational diabetes, as the name implies, is diabetes that is present only during pregnancy. Many women with gestational diabetes eventually will manifest diabetes when they are not pregnant as well. It is essential to identify the woman with gestational diabetes because this disorder represents an increased risk to both the fetus and the mother. Treatment can reduce this risk.

Women who should be considered at risk are those who:

- demonstrate glycosuria, especially on more than one occasion
- are shorter than 5'5" and weigh more than 150 pounds during or prior to the first trimester
- are taller than 5'5" and weigh more than 180 pounds during or prior to the first trimester

- have had a previous infant who weighed over 9½ pounds at birth, especially if the infant demonstrated stigmata of diabetes (e.g., generalized puffiness, plethora). It is not clear whether large size alone reflects maternal diabetes.
- have had a stillbirth
- have a family history of diabetes in parents, siblings, aunts, or uncles

Women who meet any of these criteria are advised of the importance of a one-hour 50-gm oral glucose loading test to be conducted at the 20-week visit. In addition, women with glycosuria should have a random (at least two hours after eating) or fasting glucose test performed. If the random level is equal to or greater than 120 mg/dl or the fasting level is equal to or greater than 105 mg/dl or if a two-hour postprandial level is equal to or greater than 120 mg/dl, then a three-hour glucose tolerance test should be performed instead of the glucose loading test. Further guidelines for the diagnosis and management of gestational diabetes can be found in the literature.[29-33]

Blood Pressure

The blood pressure normally varies according to a predictable pattern during pregnancy, as shown in Figure 7-1. Note the dip of 5 mm Hg systolic and diastolic below prepregnancy levels during the first and second trimesters. Thus at 20 weeks of gestation a blood pressure of 120/80, which is usually considered normal, might signify an elevated blood pressure suggestive of chronic hypertension that would be unmasked early in the third trimester. Individuals with chronic hypertension have been observed to show an exaggerated dip in blood pressure in early pregnancy, adding further diagnostic significance to "normal" readings at that time.

Traditionally, elevated blood pressure has been the sine qua non of preeclampsia. Significant blood pressure elevation has been defined as either a systolic pressure of greater than 140 mm Hg or a diastolic pressure of greater than 90 mm Hg, or as an increase of at least 30 mm Hg in the systolic pressure or at least 15 mm Hg in the diastolic pressure over prepregnancy levels.

An extensive study of the correlation between blood pressure and fetal mortality[34,35] has led some authorities to suggest a revision of the criteria for significant blood pressure elevation. Increased risk to the fetus was found when the only abnormality was a diastolic pressure of greater than 95 mm Hg. Even greater risk existed when the diastolic pressure was at least 85 mm Hg and proteinuria of 1+ or greater was also present. A new

Figure 7-1 Normal Variations in Blood Pressure During Pregnancy

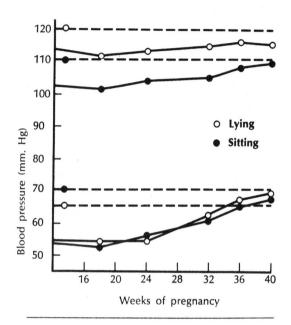

Solid lines depict mean systolic and diastolic blood pressures during normal pregnancy. The broken lines depict the mean blood pressures in normal, nonpregnant women of the same age. During the first and second trimesters, the mean systolic blood pressure is 5 mm. Hg lower and diastolic blood pressure is 10 mm. Hg lower than in the nonpregnant state. In the third trimester, blood pressure returns to nonpregnant levels.

Source: Reprinted from "The Kidney and Pregnancy," by Jeffrey P. Harris, Alexander C. Chester, and George E. Schreiner, *American Family Physician* 18, no. 4 (October 1978): 97–102. Adapted with permission from *Clinical Science and Molecular Medicine* 37 (1969): 395–407.

finding was that low maternal diastolic pressure, 65 mm Hg or less, in the third trimester was also associated with increased fetal mortality.

These more recent criteria are not too different from the traditional ones and permit an even more discriminating judgment of risk. An abnormal reading by any of these criteria should lead to the implementation of measures designed to reverse preeclampsia and is an important factor in considering whether delivery at home should be undertaken.

The reference position for blood pressure is the left lateral recumbent. An abnormal reading obtained while sitting should be checked in this position. If the reading then becomes normal, the initial finding of abnormality can be viewed as less significant.

Uterine Size

The size of the uterus is considered one of the best available indices of fetal growth. Determination of uterine size is made by stretching a measuring tape from the top of the symphysis pubis along the midline over the curve of the abdomen to the highest point of the fundus. The highest point may not be in the midline as the uterus is often tipped to one side, usually the right. The uterus should show progressive increase in size until the 36th or 38th week. Between 18 and 30 weeks, particularly in first pregnancies, the height of the uterus expressed in centimeters approximates the number of weeks of gestation. Smaller than predicted uterine growth determined over several months suggests intrauterine growth retardation or oligohydramnios (often with associated fetal anomalies) and should prompt further evaluation by uterine ultrasound. If abnormal fetal development is documented, home birth is contraindicated.

Excess uterine growth also requires an explanation. Among its causes are errors in dating the pregnancy, hydramnios, multiple pregnancy, gestational trophoblastic neoplasm, or a large baby (whether or not reflecting maternal diabetes). Ultrasonic examination is indicated to clarify the cause.

Palpation of the Fetus

During the last trimester, palpation of the fetus is part of the routine examination, one in which the couple can readily participate. Palpation has several objectives. First, the presence of more than one fetus can be suspected. Second, the size of the baby can be estimated. Third, the presentation, lie, and position of the baby can be determined.

Auscultation and Ultrasonography

The fetal heart can be auscultated by 16 to 20 weeks of gestation. When the fetal heart sounds become easy to hear, this physical finding can be shared with the couple. Extra long tubing on the fetoscope allows the woman to hear the sounds. Her partner can listen to the heart by placing his ear on her abdomen.

The fetal heartbeat can be identified with ultrasound as early as the 12th week. Thus far no harmful effects of ultrasound on the human fetus have been identified. Nevertheless, concern exists about subjecting the fetus to sound waves as a matter of routine. Parents should be informed about the costs and benefits of routine ultrasonography. The latter include more precise dating of the pregnancy and the detection of multiple pregnancy and/or congenital anomalies.

Edema

Edema (fluid accumulation in the tissues) is normal in pregnancy. Edema of the feet and legs is very common in the third trimester. It is related to increased venous pressures in the lower extremities due to pressure on the vena cava by the uterus. Many women also report that late in the day their rings are tight and their faces puffy. In traditional teaching, generalized edema (affecting other than the legs or feet) is considered an indication of increased risk, intensifies the monitoring of the pregnancy, and initiates measures to prevent preeclampsia. In one study it was shown that neither edema nor weight gain alone or in combination with other factors during the third trimester is predictive of increased fetal mortality.[36] The authors take a position between these two extremes. We regard generalized edema as a red flag to watch the pregnancy more closely for signs of preeclampsia.

While inspecting the ankles for edema, the attendant should also look for petechiae. Petechiae, which suggest platelet disorders, are most likely to appear on the ankles.

Checklist for Subsequent Prenatal Visits

The protocols given in this section for subsequent visits are summarized in Exhibit 7-3. As indicated above, visits are scheduled every four weeks until the 32nd week, at 34 and 36 weeks, and weekly thereafter.

COMMON PROBLEMS IN PREGNANCY

Sigmund Freud postulated that the discomforts of pregnancy place a woman more in touch with her own body and thus prepare her for being more sensitive to her infant's bodily needs. Pregnancy occurs during young adulthood when illness and its physical symptoms are less common than later in life. Young adults often do not have a direct experience of bodily dysfunction. They are prone to take their bodies for granted and not to be attuned to them.[37] Both partners can take advantage of the pregnancy to become more aware of their bodily functioning and how to communicate about it. Not every symptom requires medical treatment or needs relief at

Exhibit 7-3 Checklist for Subsequent Prenatal Visits

1. At each visit: blood pressure; weight; urine test for glucose and protein; measurement of fundal height (after 12 weeks); palpation of fetus (after 16 to 20 weeks); auscultation of fetal heart (after 16 to 20 weeks); appropriate physical examination according to gestational age and concerns expressed.
2. At 16 to 18 weeks: venous blood sample for screening for neural tube defects through alpha-fetoprotein determination (optional); amniocentesis as indicated.
3. At 18 to 20 weeks: glucose loading or tolerance test as indicated.
4. At 28 weeks: Rh antibody titer for Rh-negative mothers with Rh-positive partners; RhoGAM to Rh-negative antibody-negative mothers (if RhoGAM is not used, other protocols for monitoring Rh sensitization may be found in standard texts); glucose loading or tolerance test as indicated.
5. At 32 weeks: cultures for herpesvirus as indicated.
6. At 36 to 40 weeks: booklets given out on newborn care and auto safety for infants and children.
7. At 36 weeks: hematocrit and urine culture repeated; identification of back-up emergency transport and hospital; map of route to home placed in record.
8. At 37 weeks: home visit by midwife.
9. At 38 weeks: vaginal speculum examination only when indicated.
10. At 42 weeks and beyond: nonstress test weekly and 24-hour urine estriol determinations every three days; stress test as indicated. Shift to planned hospital delivery.

all costs. It is possible to endure discomfort and to become discriminating about the need for medical interventions.

Anticipating and dealing with the common problems of pregnancy is an essential part of prenatal care. General principles in responding to these problems are assessing the meaning of a symptom to the family (for example, the common fear that decreased food intake associated with morning sickness will adversely affect the fetus); speaking directly to the underlying concern; providing general information about the symptom—what is and is not known; and empathizing with the couple.

Frequency of Urination and Nocturnal Urination

Several factors are involved in increased frequency of urination. The most important is decreased bladder capacity, resulting from bladder compression by the growing uterus. Additionally, fluid retained during the day in the upright position is mobilized at night and excreted. Also contributing to increased urine output is increased intake of fluids, whether intended to relieve constipation or as part of the treatment of urinary tract infections. Frequency of urination may also reflect a urinary tract infection. When in doubt, a urine culture should be obtained.

Urinary Tract Infection

Urinary tract infection has special significance in pregnancy. The relative slowing of urine flow in pregnancy can both predispose to infection and interfere with treatment. Hence, early identification and treatment are called for. Although no preventive measures are routinely prescribed, the measures used in treatment (e.g., increased fluid intake, more frequent urination, acidification of urine with cranberry juice or vitamin C, avoidance of spicy food and caffeine) are believed to have preventive value as well.

The clinical signs of lower urinary tract infection (affecting the bladder and urethra) are urgency and frequency of urination and dysuria. Involvement of the upper tracts (affecting the ureters and kidneys) is suggested by systemic symptoms of fever, chills, nausea, vomiting, and abdominal or flank pain. Both upper and lower urinary tracts can be involved together.

Dysuria can often be identified by the patient on close questioning as "inside" the bladder or "outside" on the genitalia. The latter suggests vulvar irritation related to vaginitis, in which contact with urine is uncomfortable, and should prompt performance of a speculum examination and clinical and microscopic study of vaginal and cervical secretions. Cultures for yeast, gonococcus, or herpesvirus may also be appropriate. Treatment is specific to the identified cause.

Evaluation of urinary complaints also requires a urinalysis and urine culture. The report of typical symptoms, especially in the presence in the spun sediment of pyuria of greater than 20 white blood cells per high power field and/or bacteria of greater than 10 per high power field, argues for a presumptive diagnosis of infection and the initiation of therapy.

Most cultures taken of women who are started on treatment by these criteria will yield greater than 100,000 colonies of organisms. Growth of fewer colonies in the presence of symptoms and urinary findings as described is still consistent with infection and is not a reason for stopping treatment.

Cultures should be repeated on the third day of treatment and one week following treatment. Symptoms and signs of upper urinary tract infection should alert the attendant to a more serious problem. The oral antibiotic regimens recommended for ambulatory management may not be adequate, and the woman will usually be advised to enter the hospital for intravenous therapy.

Backache

The weight of the growing uterus stresses the lumbar spine, exaggerating its normally present lordosis, and contributes to backache in pregnancy.

Hormonal effects of pregnancy also increase ligamentous laxity. Back care, which is both preventive and curative, is emphasized in the exercise and fitness program recommended in Chapter 9. It includes attention to proper posture, learning to bend at the knees rather than at the waist, use of a firm mattress or bedboard, avoidance of obesity, use of low-heeled shoes, and abdominal strengthening exercises. Backaches developing during pregnancy are treated by a combination of rest, local heat, exercise and physical therapy, and intensification of the preventive program.

Morning Sickness

The cause of the common anorexia, nausea, and vomiting of the first trimester is not fully understood. Hormonal influences are believed to play a major role, although proof for this hypothesis is lacking. There is no evidence to indicate that the decreased food intake associated with morning sickness is harmful to the fetus, a fact that should be reassuring. Measures that have been proven helpful in relieving the symptom, more by experience than by research, are eating small, frequent meals, e.g., six per day; separating the ingestion of liquids and solids by one-half hour; taking a dry unsalted cracker or biscuit before getting out of bed in the morning; and using the vitamin pyridoxine, 40 to 100 mg daily. Another drug that was available until 1983 was Bendectin®, which, despite FDA approval and the lack of persuasive evidence that it was a source of teratogenesis, was voluntarily withdrawn by the manufacturer because of controversy (including litigation) over fetal damage.

Severe nausea and vomiting in early pregnancy suggest gestational trophoblastic neoplasm. Nonpregnancy-related causes such as brain tumor and intestinal obstruction also need to be excluded. Only after eliminating known causes of severe hyperemesis can the diagnosis of hyperemesis gravidarum be entertained. This is a serious disorder of unknown cause that usually requires hospital care to prevent maternal death.

Pain in Lower Abdomen and Thighs

Pain in the lower quadrants of the abdomen, especially on the right side, is common in pregnancy and is believed to be due to stretching of uterine supports, especially the round ligaments. Verification of this plausible hypothesis seems almost impossible. The pain emanating from uterine supports, the "round ligament syndrome," usually occurs at about 20 weeks of gestation and must be distinguished from the pain arising from appendicitis, cholecystitis, ureteral colic, urinary tract infection, or hernia. The pain stemming from the supporting structures of the uterus should be related to position and usually is reduced when the woman lies on the painful side or is recumbent. It is not normally associated with fever, anorexia, nausea, vomiting, diarrhea, or urinary symptoms. On physical examination there are no signs of peritoneal irritation such as guarding, spasm, or rebound tenderness. Most women are able to accept stretching pain as long as they know that it does not represent a threat either to themselves or their babies. Pain or paresthesia in the upper anterior thigh is believed to be due to pressure of the fetal presenting part on the sensory nerve that supplies the thigh as it loops over the pelvic brim. The resulting discomfort can be explained as similar to that experienced in an ulnar nerve paresthesia. It can often be relieved in the supine or lateral recumbent position, especially on the side of the pain. It does not persist after delivery.

The diagnosis of appendicitis in pregnancy can be problematic. First, anorexia, nausea, and vomiting in pregnancy are common. Second, the enlarging uterus commonly displaces the appendix upward out of its usual position in the right lower abdomen. Third, some elevation in the white blood cell count is common in pregnancy. A high index of suspicion is required if this diagnosis is to be made early, prior to rupture of the appendix.

Pain in the pelvic girdle late in pregnancy and a "coming apart" feeling can be related to the loosening of the ligaments that join the various pelvic bones. This loosening has the positive value of allowing the pelvis to "give" during the passage of the baby through the birth canal and is a counterpoint to the molding of the baby's head made possible by the open cranial sutures. There is no specific treatment for this ligament laxity other than the avoidance of strenuous activities that can intensify the strain. The rare problem of frank separation of the symphysis pubis is dealt with through strapping.

Hair Loss

Hair loss, which is almost always temporary, is one of the most distressing developments in the birth process. It results from premature cessation of growth in certain hair follicles. This conversion from the growing (anagen) to the resting (telogen) state resembles normal hair follicle behavior at the end of a growth cycle. Diffuse hair shedding during combing may occur within three months of delivery. Diagnostic protocols are available to identify the occasional case of pathological hair loss in pregnancy.[38]

The common occurrence of a telogen effluvium (in varying degrees) in the postpartum period can be explained to the couple. The same phenomenon occurs in the newborn and accounts for the shedding of the hair (lanugo) present at birth. A woman can anticipate return of shed hair within one year of delivery.

Constipation

Less frequent, harder, and more difficult to pass stools are common in pregnancy. Contributing factors are slowed intestinal peristalsis, resulting in increased resorption of water, and pressure on the rectum by the presenting part. Hemorrhoids may intensify and in turn be intensified by constipation. Constipation usually can be alleviated by increased fluid intake (which, however, contributes to another source of discomfort—frequent urination), increased fiber intake (e.g., raw fruit and vegetables, bran, psyllium seeds), and exercise. A gentle laxative such as milk of magnesia may be used as necessary. Stool softeners (e.g., diocytl sodium sulfo-succinate) are also useful.

Lactose intolerance increases in adulthood. Increased milk consumption in pregnancy can lead to an alternating cycle of constipation and diarrhea. Lact-Aid can make it possible for the woman to drink milk without these disturbances.

Varicose Veins

Varicose veins of the legs, rectum (hemorrhoids), and vulva are common in pregnancy, particularly in women with positive family histories of this disorder. Pressure of the gravid uterus on the inferior vena cava is a primary factor, intensified by the force of gravity in the upright position. Leg varicosities are primarily of cosmetic significance, although some individuals may complain of aching. Rectal varicosities can bleed and form painful fissures.

Symptomatic leg varicosities can be relieved through elevation of the legs and the use of elastic stockings. Hemorrhoids are treated by measures to prevent constipation (as listed above), sitz baths in warm water, lubricating creams, suppositories (witch hazel, Anusol®), and avoidance of straining at stool (what the English have called an "unhurried motion"). The woman can look forward to relief from varicosities following delivery even though hemorrhoids may be more pronounced in labor and the postpartum period. Because of this expected postpartum improvement, considerations of surgical correction should be delayed if at all possible. Thrombosis of an external hemorrhoid can be very painful; its clot can be removed by excising an elliptical segment of overlying skin. If bleeding is persistent or if the hemorrhoids are reducible or infected, hemorrhoidectomy may be required. Ligation or injection is preferred over more radical approaches. Varicosities of the vulva may be contained and relieved with counterpressure by a foam rubber pad held with a belt of the kind used with a perineal pad.

Leg Cramps

Many pregnant women have calf cramps. Speculation has related these to calcium deficiency, excess phosphate intake, or excessive milk consumption. Treatment includes changing the source of calcium by decreasing milk consumption, taking 1 gm calcium lactate per day, or increasing the intake of green vegetables, sesame seeds, tofu and other soy products, or other dietary sources of calcium. Physical measures include massage and stretching maneuvers with dorsiflexion of the foot.

Lightening

"Lightening" is the subjective sensation experienced by a woman as the presenting part descends during the latter weeks of pregnancy. It is not the same as engagement, which refers to the passage of the largest diameter of the presenting part through the pelvic inlet. Symptoms of lightening include less shortness of breath; decreased epigastric pressure; a feeling that the baby has "dropped"; increased pressure in the pelvis; increased backache, urinary frequency, and constipation; initial appearance or aggravation of hemorrhoids and varicose veins of the legs; edema of the legs and feet; and increased difficulty in walking.

Heartburn

Heartburn is a common problem in pregnancy and reflects reflux of gastric contents into the esophagus. Contributing factors are compression of the abdominal viscera (including the stomach) by the enlarging uterus, elevation of the stomach, alterations in the gastroesophageal sphincter, and relaxation of smooth muscle in the gastrointestinal tract.

This symptom can be prevented in large part by eating smaller quantities at a time, not lying down immediately after eating, and, if these measures fail, using antacids at the end of each meal. For symptoms present on retiring, elevating the head of the bed six to eight inches with blocks beneath the bed posts allows gravity to work against reflux.

Multiple Pregnancy

In a home birth practice the identification of multiple pregnancy is crucial because of increased risk to both fetus and mother. The authors regard multiple pregnancy as a contraindication to home birth. Multiple pregnancy can easily be overlooked. Its clinical signs are often not clear cut. Clinical findings that are suggestive include uterine size large for dates, report by the woman of fetal activity throughout her abdomen, palpation of more than two fetal poles, and determination of more than one fetal heart as documented by the observation of two or more different heart rates through simultaneous auscultation at two sites by two observers. The suspicion of multiple pregnancy warrants an ultrasound examination.

Preeclampsia

Preeclampsia is said to exist when hypertension develops, along with proteinuria or edema or both, after the 20th week of gestation. Hypertension is defined as an increase in blood pressure to greater than 140 mm Hg systolic or greater than 90 mm Hg diastolic (or 84 mm Hg diastolic with at least 1+ proteinuria), or an increase of greater than 30 mm Hg systolic or 15 mm Hg diastolic over the prepregnancy level. (Blood pressure of 140/90 or greater at the onset of pregnancy suggests chronic hypertension, which in itself contraindicates home birth.) Together with hypertension, proteinuria of 2+ or greater that is not corrected by position is indicative of preeclampsia, as is generalized edema. It should be noted, however, that edema in pregnancy occurs more often in the absence of preeclampsia than in association with it. Traditionally, weight gain of more than two pounds in one week has been viewed as characteristic of preeclampsia. This view has been challenged. (All four factors mentioned here have been discussed previously in the section on subsequent prenatal visits.)

Occurrence of the symptoms and signs of preeclampsia prior to the 20th week suggests gestational trophoblastic neoplasm. Other findings suggestive of this disorder are vaginal bleeding (most common), excessive increase in uterine size, and high chorionic gonadotropin levels. The reader is referred to standard obstetric texts for further discussion.

When the symptoms of headache, blurred vision, and abdominal pain and the finding of hyperactive deep tendon reflexes are present, preeclampsia should be considered severe, with immediate hospitalization indicated. For milder forms of preeclampsia a program that is sometimes effective can be initiated at home and in the office. The elements of this program are listed below:

- resting on the left side for one-hour periods at least twice a day in midmorning and midafternoon when the woman is normally upright
- increasing fluid intake by 8 to 10 glasses of liquid per day (preferably water)

- increasing daily protein intake (e.g., by 2 tablespoons of brewer's yeast or 3 to 6 eggs) in the context of adequate calories
- eliminating added salt in cooking or at the table and avoiding salt-rich foods
- checking blood pressure and urine protein at least once daily, measurements that can be made at home by the midwife or by the couple

It should be noted, however, that the added fluids and protein have never been proven to be effective despite their popularity. Above all, the attendants and the family should be alert to the potential for rapid deterioration and therefore to the importance of careful monitoring and adherence to the measures specified above even when the mother appears to be doing well.

In general, the diagnosis of preeclampsia precludes a home birth. However, there are very mild cases that respond quickly to the measures listed, and there is room for individual judgment in such situations. In an illustrative case from the authors' practice, a woman with elevated blood pressure (maximum 160/105) and florid edema was able to reverse this preeclamptic presentation and achieve an uneventful home birth two weeks later after a week of normal blood pressure and loss of edema.

Herpesvirus Infection

Herpesvirus infection of the newborn can be a serious, life-threatening disease. At present, treatment is only partially effective. With rare exceptions, the virus is contracted by the infant during its passage through the birth canal from lesions on the mother's genitalia. Prevention of contact between the infant and virus can be accomplished most effectively through cesarean section, assuming that the membranes have not been ruptured for more than four to six hours.

If either the woman or her partner has a history of genital herpes, it is recommended that viral cultures of the cervix be taken at 32, 34, and 36 weeks of gestation and weekly thereafter. Less accurate than cultures in detecting infection (about 75 percent effective) are Papanicolaou smears of the cervix, which can identify multinucleated giant cells stimulated by viral infection.

A woman is considered to be not infected and still a candidate for vaginal delivery if results of virological and/or cytological studies are negative on two successive examinations, the last of which is obtained within one week before delivery, and if clinical lesions are not detected during labor.

If the partner has a documented genital infection, avoidance of genital contact in the last several months of pregnancy is recommended. If the partner has "cold sores" of the mouth (type 1 herpesvirus), oral-genital sex should also be avoided since herpesvirus type 1 can also infect the genitalia and is transmissible to the infant.

The recommendations given here for choosing between vaginal delivery and cesarean section in cases in which herpesvirus is or has been present, which are based on two reviews,[39,40] are summarized in Table 7-3.

After birth, mothers or other family members with cold sores of the mouth should not kiss or nuzzle the newborn. They should cover the lesions if exposed and should wash their hands prior to handling the infant.

ASPECTS OF PRENATAL CARE IN LATE PREGNANCY

Pelvic Examination

The practice of routinely performing a vaginal examination between the 37th and 39th weeks is no longer recommended, since the examination does not yield information sufficiently useful to justify the increased incidence of premature rupture of the membranes. The examination should be performed selectively in consultation with the family, as when a discharge raises suspicion of a pathological condition, or when herpesvirus is suspected.

External Version of Breech

Because of the increased risk associated with breech presentations and the inadvisability of delivering a breech infant at home, it is desirable to attempt to convert breech to vertex presentations prior to the onset of labor. There are two ways to achieve this conversion: (1) by maternal positioning and (2) by external cephalic version.

The maternal positioning method involves the mother's lying supine on a hard surface with her buttocks elevated on a pillow for 10 to 20 minutes three to four times a day after the 30th week for up to four weeks or until version occurs, whichever is earlier. To the authors' knowledge the success rate of this maneuver has not been studied carefully. Anecdotally it appears to be effective.

The second method of conversion involves the attendants' rotating the baby manually. The expected success rate of this maneuver after the 37th week is about 70 percent. Before the 37th week there is a higher reversion rate; hence, 37 weeks is considered the optimal time for the procedure. The risk of the procedure's interfering with the blood supply to the fetus is not well defined. Many obstetricians nonetheless advise against this

Table 7-3 Recommendations for Cesarean Section At Term in Women with Prior or Concurrent Herpes

Genital herpetic lesions present at birth	Group	Primary genital lesions	Recurrent genital lesions (or genital reinfection)	Status of membranes*	Recommended route of delivery†
Yes	1	+		Intact or ruptured <4–6 hours	Cesarean section
	2	+		Ruptured >4–6 hours	Vaginal
	3	+	or +	Baby has been delivered vaginally	
	4		+	Intact or ruptured <4–6 hours	Cesarean section
	5		+	Ruptured >4–6 Hours	Vaginal
No, but cervicovaginal culture or cytology is positive for herpesvirus	6			Intact or ruptured <4–6 hours	Cesarean section
	7			Ruptured >4–6 hours	Vaginal
No, but there is past history of genital herpesvirus, presently inactive or status unknown	8			Intact or ruptured	Vaginal
No, but nongenital herpesvirus is present at term	9			Intact or ruptured	Vaginal
No, but there is past history of nongenital herpesvirus	10			Intact or ruptured	Vaginal

*The shorter the interval between rupture of the membranes and cesarean section, the less is the risk of fetal infection. The critical period appears to be four to six hours.
†Dependent on evaluation of individual risks and benefits.

Source: Reprinted from "Herpes Simplex Infection at Term: What to Do With Mother, Newborn, and Nursery Personnel," by Sidney Kibrick, *Journal of the American Medical Association* 243 (1980): 157–160. © 1980, American Medical Association.

procedure. It is conceivable that such interference could be fatal to the infant. How often such an outcome occurs is not known. This potential risk should be shared with the woman and her partner. Any evidence of impaired fetal well-being as determined by the fetal heart rate is considered an indication for immediately repositioning the fetus in the breech presentation.

External version should be done by or under the supervision of an experienced attendant. The breech must not be engaged in the pelvis. Some clinicians require prior placental localization by ultrasound and avoid the procedure in anteriorly positioned placentas to avoid placental abruption.[41] In some settings the version is carried out only in the hospital using intravenous terbutaline to relax the uterus and thereby facilitate the maneuver. The authors do not insist on either of these requirements.

The fetal heart rate is determined at the beginning and end of the procedure. Some clinicians suggest checking the rate midway through the procedure as well. Marked increase or decrease or irregularity in the heart rate is considered a sign of fetal distress and an indication for repositioning the fetus.

The fetus is turned through the shorter of the two possible arcs so that the head takes the shortest route to the pelvis. Following a successful version the woman is asked to stay in the upright position for the rest of the day. The version may be repeated once if necessary. In the authors' practice, failure to maintain the vertex position after two versions following the 37th week is considered a contraindication to further efforts. Rh-negative women with Rh-positive partners should be given RhoGAM after an attempted version.

Discussion of Labor

Late in the third trimester the agreements made at the outset of the pregnancy regarding the management of labor (including such sensitive issues as analgesic medications and decision-making authority when prompt intervention is required) are reaffirmed. Particularly in a first pregnancy, the intense, difficult-to-anticipate quality of labor pain is acknowledged, along with the feeling commonly expressed by women in labor as well as their partners that they "can't go on." The attendants outline the kind of guidance and support they will provide (described in Chapter 11) to help the couple complete their intended home birth in spite of such normal feelings of discouragement and exhaustion. The course of labor as a woman experiences it is reviewed, and the retrospective accounts of many women on the value of the experience of normal labor, in spite of the pain, are cited. The attendants make clear that they will be alert to any signs of failure of progress, physical or psychological collapse on the part of the mother, or fetal distress. On the strength of the trusting relationship that has developed in the course of the pregnancy, the woman and her partner are assured that the attendants will speak the truth about what is happening and will know when the woman really "can't make it."

Vitamin K

By the 38th week the couple is presented with information regarding vitamin K prophylaxis of blood clotting abnormalities in the newborn. Traditionally, vitamin K has been administered to the infant in its vitamin K_1 form (phytonadione [AquaMEPHYTON®]). Stimulated by concerned parents who want to avoid a painful injection for their infant, some practitioners give phytonadione to the newborn either by mouth, 1.0 to 2.0 mg,[42] or via the placenta prenatally by having the mother take 5 to 10 mg vitamin K_1 daily beginning 14 days preceding the estimated date of birth and continuing until birth.[43]

Prophylaxis of Gonococcal Eye Infection

All states mandate treatment of the newborn's eyes to prevent gonococcal infection. Some states follow the standards of the Centers for Disease Control in allowing a choice among silver nitrate, erythromycin ointment (0.5 percent), and tetracycline ointment (1 percent). The two antibiotic ointments have been shown to be effective against gonococcal and the even more common chlamydial conjunctivitis.[44] Other states restrict treatment to the traditional use of silver nitrate solution. Many parents have objected to the use of silver nitrate on the grounds that the swelling of the conjunctivae and lids that commonly results interferes with the infant's ability to open its eyes and thereby inhibits parent-infant bonding, an important ingredient of which is eye contact.[45]

Map and Medical Record

The attendants should request and place in the medical record a map with directions to the home. It may be advisable for the couple to have a copy of the medical record to bring to the hospital as needed.

Home Visit

It is advisable for the midwife to make a home visit at 37 to 38 weeks of gestation. This is the only home visit prior to labor. Its purposes are several: learning where the home is; affirming in the family's mind the intention of the attendants to come to the home for the birth as agreed; observing the physical layout of the birthing room; discussing procedures and concerns; meeting other participants, dramatizing that the caregivers are guests of the family; and celebrating with the family the accomplishment of the pregnancy.

Inquiry should be made into the arrangements made by the couple for transfer to hospital should this be necessary. The couple may be asked to identify two nearby ambulance services that are willing to provide such transport. The phone numbers of these services should be readily accessible in the home.

The home visit is an ideal opportunity to assess how responsibly a given family is preparing for home birth. Being responsible about birth begins with being responsible about prenatal care, which includes punctuality for appointments and class sessions, forthrightness with attendants, and adherence to agreed-on nutritional guidelines, all of which will have become apparent by the time of the home visit. It also includes preparation of the home (e.g., supplies ready, emergency transportation arranged, the home reasonably orderly and functional). Given the personal growth that can occur so remarkably during pregnancy, a mature attitude may emerge more strongly as the birth draws near.

If there are any questions about a couple's attitude, they should be aired thoroughly with the couple. Some families need encouragement to see themselves as competent to make responsible choices, especially when their parents or friends may be calling them irresponsible for choosing home birth. Families who deny that there are any risks to their choice need to be confronted forcefully with the reality of uncertainty and the potential for a grave outcome. Families who look to the attendant for direction and protection in an immature, dependent way need to be informed of the limits of the attendant's role. If these issues cannot be resolved, the home birth should be reconsidered.

Pregnancies That Go Beyond the Estimated Date of Birth

On a statistical basis, pregnancies that exceed 42 weeks of gestation by estimated dates are at higher risk for fetal malnutrition, the syndrome of placental insufficiency and dysmaturity. Affected infants are at increased risk for death both prior to and during labor, for illness in the newborn period, and for later developmental abnormalities. It is therefore desirable to identify such infants prior to labor. They are considered to be at high risk and should be delivered in the hospital where electronic fetal monitoring and prompt access to surgical intervention and neonatal and intensive-care facilities are available. At present, the best screening tests for identifying such infants are the nonstress test, stress test, and urinary estriol levels. As indicated in Chapter 5, however, the authors' policy, regardless of the test results, is to plan for a hospital delivery.

NOTES

1. Stanley E. Sagov with Archie Brodsky, *The Active Patient's Guide to Better Medical Care* (New York: McKay, 1976).

2. Harold Bursztajn et al., *Medical Choices, Medical Chances: How Patients, Families, and Physicians Can Cope With Uncertainty* (New York: Delacorte Press/Seymour Lawrence, 1981), pp. 349–388.

3. Aubrey Milunsky, *Know Your Genes* (Boston: Houghton Mifflin, 1977).

4. Stephen G. Pauker and Susan B. Pauker, "Decision Making in the Practice of Medicine," in Percy H. Hill et al. (eds.), *Making Decisions: A Multidisciplinary Introduction* (Reading, Mass.: Addison-Wesley, 1978), pp. 152–176.

5. Susan Perlmutter Pauker and Stephen G. Pauker, "The Amniocentesis Decision: An Explicit Guide for Parents," *Birth Defects: Original Article Series* 15 (1979): 289–324.

6. J.M. Bowman and J.M. Pollock, "Antenatal Prophylaxis of Rh Isoimmunization: 28 Weeks'-Gestation Service Program," *Canadian Medical Association Journal* 118 (1978): 627–630.

7. Calvin M. Kunin, *Detection, Prevention, and Management of Urinary Tract Infections,* 3rd ed. (Philadelphia: Lea & Febiger, 1979), pp. 44–45.

8. Richard L. Naeye, "Causes of the Excessive Rates of Perinatal Mortality and Prematurity in Pregnancies Complicated by Maternal Urinary-Tract Infections," *New England Journal of Medicine* 300 (1979): 819–823.

9. Robert E. Harris, "The Significance of Eradication of Bacteriuria During Pregnancy," *Obstetrics and Gynecology* 53 (1979): 71–73.

10. James N. Macri and Robert R. Weiss, "α-Fetoprotein Screening for Neural Tube Defects," *Obstetrics and Gynecology* 59 (1982): 633–639.

11. James A. Krick and Jack S. Remington, "Toxoplasmosis in the Adult—An Overview," *New England Journal of Medicine* 298 (1978): 550–553.

12. Jeffrey J. Freitag and Leslie W. Miller (eds.), *Manual of Medical Therapeutics,* 23rd ed. (Boston: Little, Brown, 1980), pp. 452–454.

13. Katherine Tennes and Carol Blackard, "Maternal Alcohol Consumption, Birth Weight, and Minor Physical Anomalies," *American Journal of Obstetrics and Gynecology* 138 (1980): 774–780.

14. David U. Himmelberger, Byron W. Brown, Jr., and Ellis N. Cohen, "Cigarette Smoking During Pregnancy and the Occurrence of Spontaneous Abortion and Congenital Abnormality," *American Journal of Epidemiology* 108 (1978): 470–479.

15. Susan Harlap and A. Michael Davies, "Infant Admissions to Hospital and Maternal Smoking," *Lancet* 1 (1974): 529–532.

16. Stanley M. Garn, "Tell Pregnant Patients: Do *Not* Smoke!" *Medical Times* 108, no. 10 (October 1980): 18s–30s.

17. Richard L. Naeye, "Abruptio Placentae and Placenta Previa: Frequency, Perinatal Mortality, and Cigarette Smoking," *Obstetrics and Gynecology* 55 (1980): 701–704.

18. Robert M. Kretzschmar, "Smoking and Health: The Role of the Obstetrician and Gynecologist," *Obstetrics and Gynecology* 55 (1980): 403–406.

19. Richard L. Naeye, "Coitus and Associated Amniotic Fluid Infections," *New England Journal of Medicine* 301 (1979): 1198–1200.

20. Emanuel A. Friedman and Raymond K. Neff, *Pregnancy Hypertension: A Systematic Evaluation of Clinical Diagnostic Criteria* (Littleton, Mass.: PSG Publishing, 1977), pp. 29–175.

21. Emanuel A. Friedman and Raymond K. Neff, "Hypertension-Hypotension in Pregnancy: Correlation With Fetal Outcome," *Journal of the American Medical Association* 239 (1978): 2249–2251.

22. Richard L. Naeye, "Weight Gain and the Outcome of Pregnancy," *American Journal of Obstetrics and Gynecology* 135 (1979): 3–9.

23. Helen Varney, *Nurse-Midwifery* (Boston: Blackwell Scientific Publications, 1980), pp. 125–129.

24. Bernice K. Watt et al., *Handbook of the Nutritional Contents of Foods* (New York: Dover Publications, 1975).

25. Nikki Goldbeck, *As You Eat So Your Baby Grows* (Woodstock, N.Y.: Ceres Press, 1977).

26. Friedman and Neff, *Pregnancy Hypertension,* p. 237.

27. Jeffrey P. Harris, Alexander C. Chester, and George E. Schreiner, "The Kidney and Pregnancy," *American Family Physician* 18, no. 4 (October 1978): 97–102.

28. Ibid., pp. 97–102.

29. Kofi S. Amankwah, "Screening for Gestational Diabetes by Plasma Glucose Levels," *American Journal of Obstetrics and Gynecology* 126 (1976): 1052.

30. American Diabetes Association Workshop—Conference on Gestational Diabetes, "Summary and Recommendations," *Diabetes Care* 3 (1980): 499–501.

31. John B. O'Sullivan et al., "Screening Criteria for High-Risk Gestational Diabetic Patients," *American Journal of Obstetrics and Gynecology* 116 (1973): 895–900.

32. John B. O'Sullivan et al., "Medical Treatment of the Gestational Diabetic," *Obstetrics and Gynecology* 43 (1974): 817–821.

33. Ibid.

34. Friedman and Neff, *Pregnancy Hypertension,* pp. 238–239.

35. Friedman and Neff, "Hypertension-Hypotension in Pregnancy." pp. 2249–2251.

36. Friedman and Neff, *Pregnancy Hypertension,* p. 238.

37. Stanley E. Sagov, "The Young Adult," in Robert B. Taylor (ed.), *Family Medicine: Principles and Practice* (New York: Springer-Verlag, 1978), pp. 173–190.

38. Willard D. Steck, "The Clinical Evaluation of Pathologic Hair Loss With a Diagnostic Sign in Trichotillomania," *Cutis* 24 (1979): 293–301.

39. Sidney Kibrick, "Herpes Simplex Infection at Term: What to Do With Mother, Newborn, and Nursery Personnel," *Journal of the American Medical Association* 243 (1980): 157–160.

40. Committee on Fetus and Newborn, Committee on Infectious Diseases, American Academy of Pediatrics, "Perinatal Herpes Simplex Virus Infections," *Pediatrics* 66 (1980): 147–148.

41. Ole Fall and Bo A. Nilsson, "External Cephalic Version in Breech Presentation Under Tocolysis," *Obstetrics and Gynecology* 53 (1979): 712–715.

42. Committee on Nutrition, American Academy of Pediatrics, "Vitamin K Compounds and the Water-Soluble Analogues: Use in Therapy and Prophylaxis in Pediatrics," *Pediatrics* 28 (1961): 501–507.

43. George M. Owen et al., "Use of Vitamin K_1 in Pregnancy," *American Journal of Obstetrics and Gynecology* 99 (1967): 368–373.

44. Margaret R. Hammerschlag et al., "Erythromycin Ointment for Ocular Prophylaxis of Neonatal Chlamydial Infection," *Journal of the American Medical Association* 244 (1980): 2291–2293.

45. Vivian Wahlbert et al., "Reconsideration of Credé Prophylaxis: A Study of Maternity and Neonatal Care," *Acta Paediatrica Scandinavica* Supplement 295 (1982): 1–73.

Chapter 8

Childbirth Education

Principal Authors: Jenifer M. Fleming and Peggy Spindel, R.N.

Since home birth is not a mainstream choice in the United States, those making this choice are vulnerable to feelings of isolation. Sometimes these families realize the extent of their isolation only when they notice the relief they feel on meeting others who are likewise deviating from the norm. It is painful to lose, at such a ritually significant time as the birth of a child, strong cultural identification of the sort that once supported home birth in America and Europe and still does in the Netherlands.[1] Childbirth education oriented to the home is a vehicle for building new rituals and new cultural ties.

Both the birth and learning processes have a paradoxical quality, in that, while one seeks as much information as possible, one increasingly becomes aware of instinctual skills already possessed. People bring to childbirth, and to childbirth education, fears (of failure, of pain, of death) as well as confidence (in their abilities and strengths, in the drive of the natural process to make new life). Likewise, a woman in labor wants to be in control but knows that nature will take its course. Families and attendants try to choose an intelligent risk/safety balance even while aware that the universe does not always honor human choice. The childbirth educator worries whether the discussion of possible negative outcomes will increase or decrease fear (and which is the more appropriate goal for a particular family). If one is to acknowledge the reality of both the joy and the fear, one must seek to embrace rather than resolve the paradoxes.

The educator must help couples develop tools to deal with uncertainty, to weigh choices and make decisions, with the understanding that prediction is a matter of probability rather than absolute certainty.[2] (There is also no certainty in the hospital, but people who have home births must take greater responsibility for risks, since the particular risks they have chosen are not supported by society.) Where does one turn when there are no guarantees? Slowly couples come to realize that they can influence the odds. They begin to understand that how they deal with the past and how well they live in the present have a concrete bearing on the future.

Pregnancy and birth then become an educational opportunity. Birth can be a significant threshold not only for a new individual life but also for all whom the birth touches.[3] Families can improve their nutrition, exercise habits, stress management skills, and quality of communication and decision making. Children and friends of the family educate themselves about elemental aspects of human life. New relationships and traditions form.

Changing body images and changing self-perceptions make pregnant women particularly open to learning. Families are engaged in women's acts of generation. It is not only babies that grow.

A NEW MODEL OF CHILDBIRTH EDUCATION

On a midsummer's evening a group of eight couples in late pregnancy gathered in the living room of a house in Cambridge, Massachusetts, with a childbirth educator and her assistant. There was an air of merriment and gaiety as the women joked about how big they had grown and how many refreshments they were going to eat that night. There was also a spirit of community among these men and women, strangers to one another eight weeks earlier, who now were about to complete their last childbirth preparation class.

While anticipating new life, these 16 people had talked of unexpected deaths of mothers and infants; they had talked of hospitals, physicians, midwives, and circumstances of birth beyond their control; they had seen and heard slides, films, and tapes of births; they had pondered the issue of circumcision and grappled with family conflicts surrounding their impending births. Much of a very intimate nature had been shared: fears, worries, dreams, and fantasies.

There was an air of celebration, a celebration of how much the classes and the experience of pregnancy had meant to each person present. It was one man's birthday, and he and his wife had volunteered to bring the snack that night. Lights were turned low and a hush came over the room as the couple came in bearing a large cake with eight candles. A man at the piano struck up "Happy Birthday"—a double-entendre, since the name of the childbirth education group was Birth Day. The man whose birthday was being celebrated spoke quietly of how much the classes had given him and how each of the participants had contributed to his own growth and understanding of birth, life, and death. He reached for his guitar and, with his captive audience alternately laughing and crying, sang two songs he had just written: "How Will We Know," a song about the beginnings of labor, and "The Late Baby Blues," about waiting for labor to begin.

For these 16 "strangers," the eight weeks of childbirth education classes had done more than transmit information about the physiology of labor and birth. They had stimulated mutuality, creativity, vision, and inspiration. The obstetrician Michel Odent, in a lecture in Boston in 1980, described his work as a childbirth educator in Pithiviers, France, in these words: "We gather together pregnant and postpartum couples around the grand piano in our center, and we sing, joke, and share birthing stories."[4] In Odent's center, people whose birth practices are regarded as unusual and even deviant give one another invaluable support. The spirit in that living room in Cambridge was similar to that which Odent described at Pithiviers. It is a spirit that gives couples a positive attitude toward birth and enables them to recognize, accept, and finally transcend their fears and concerns while preparing for complications that may arise.

This is not standard childbirth education. Rather, it is a model of what childbirth education can be. Of the many varieties of childbirth education courses available, some have offered little more than a stamp of approval for hospital practices then in vogue. In many classes a preoccupation with details of anatomy and physiology and an advocacy of elaborate and often contrived breathing techniques lead women to lose faith in the normal and natural process of birth. Women look to such techniques, as propounded by "the experts," to guide and direct them through the experience of birth, instead of trusting the normal physiology of their bodies and their own and their partners' inner strengths. In this standard model, childbirth instructors have seen themselves as "aiding" the health care system rather than enabling parents to reevaluate traditional methods and assumptions.

In part as a result of the shortcomings of this kind of childbirth education, groups have arisen in many parts of the country specifically to meet the educational needs of couples planning home births. Some groups have been initiated by childbirth instructors disillusioned with conventional approaches. Others have been formed by parents concerned with exploring new ways of handling birth outside the hospital.

The Boston-based organization called Birth Day developed in the early 1970s and has evolved steadily since then. Started by couples together with a few nurses concerned about birthing alternatives, the group met in one another's homes to share experiences, question possible options, and seek alternatives. It was a support group of people who wanted to educate themselves and the public about ways of birthing. Its purposes were articulated in the following statement, written in 1973:

> Birth Day exists because there are women and men who want to seek out the form of their own birthing, to reclaim the birth experience as their own, and who want to make it possible for

others to do the same. Birth Day exists to promote and protect the normal in our births, wherever those births occur, at home, in a hospital or in a maternity home. The meaning of Birth Day continues to evolve as we grow in our understanding of what birth can be when there is no unnecessary interference, and as we explore the relationship of birth to our total lives.

Today Birth Day offers a series of eight prenatal classes and one post-partum class in four areas of metropolitan Boston. The classes are oriented toward home birth but are also attended by couples who plan alternative births in the hospital. There is a maximum of eight couples in each series (single parents are encouraged to bring a friend throughout). Each series is led by a woman carefully selected for her sensitivity, alertness, flexibility, ease with herself and her experiences, and openness to self-criticism and growth. (In this discussion it is assumed that childbirth educators are women, although classes may also be co-led by couples.) Prospective teachers go through a training program in which they learn by observation, apprenticeship, and supervised experience. The Birth Day classes are the model for the recommendations in this chapter.

CONTEXTS OF CHILDBIRTH EDUCATION

Childbirth education is not limited to the classes conducted for that purpose. Many couples inform themselves through reading and informal discussion with other families. Professional birth attendants teach in the course of giving prenatal care. The birth experience itself is an educational one. Although the discussion in this chapter emphasizes childbirth classes, the substance of childbirth education is in practice conveyed through all of these channels.

Self-Education

When women teach themselves and each other about birth, teaching and learning have an informal, spontaneous quality. Even under more formal circumstances, teaching is most effective (and efficient) when the woman has done some reading on her own or at least given some thought to her concerns and needs only guidance to structure her choices. To this end, self-education can be encouraged by informing families of various sources of information such as seminars or classes; by discussing and recommending books (maintaining a lending library, referring families to good bookstores); and by introducing families who live near each other or share common interests.

Role of Birth Attendants

Prenatal care is an educational process as well as one of health screening. As a rule, midwives have more time than physicians to be childbirth educators. All professionals should, however, be conscious of their educational role, which may be more or less crucial depending on the adequacy of the childbirth classes available in a given locality.

In addition to providing direct instruction, the attendant can take the following steps to encourage women to educate each other and build a community of awareness about birth:

- Provide a physical space that can be used as an informal meeting place for families. An office with a large waiting room (or adjoining room) or a birth center with meeting space might be offered if community groups do not have space of their own. Books, toys, a bulletin board, and ample seating capacity will contribute to making people feel welcome.
- Share knowledge and teach skills to families. A woman can do much of her own prenatal screening,[5] and family members can give her much of the support she needs in labor. Parents can learn to do health screening for themselves and their children (e.g., throat cultures).[6] Self-help groups are ongoing in many large cities and should be encouraged by professionals (e.g., Couple-to-Couple League for natural family planning, local women's self-help groups).
- Participate in the life of the community as an individual and as a family. Much spontaneous teaching can take place when a home birth attendant gets to know clients and prospective clients as neighbors, if not as intimate friends. By using child care services offered by families in the community (perhaps in exchange for health care), the attendant meets women, instructs them, and learns from them.

The Experience of Birth

Home birth itself is an excellent educational experience for those present. If enough children, adolescents, and young adults participate in births, the daughters and sons of today's home birth couples may not be dependent on childbirth classes when they bear children.

Childbirth Classes

Childbirth classes provide a format for transmitting any necessary information that women and their partners do not receive from the other sources listed here. They also provide much more, namely, an experience of mutual learning and a forum for discussion of issues and feelings that is independent of the client-attendant relationship.

GUIDELINES FOR CHILDBIRTH TEACHING

The following are basic guidelines for teachers who lead childbirth classes. They are all interdependent and of equal importance.

Building Group Feeling

The purpose of the classes is not just to impart reliable information about physiology, nutrition, exercise, and relaxation but also to support the people in the group and to enable them to support one another as people are thought to have done in the old-fashioned village community. The instructor can help build group feeling in the following ways:

The instructor introduces herself at the beginning of the series by describing her own birth choices and interests, thereby giving others permission to speak openly about theirs.

The first class includes a round robin of introductions and open-ended questions to draw people out, such as "Why did you choose this childbirth class?" "What are your expectations from the class?" "What do you plan for your birth?"

A 15-minute break for snack and socializing is scheduled for every class. Each family, by bringing the food for one session, gets an added feeling of contributing to the group. If the food table is placed where people have to get up and mingle, issues may be raised there that can be taken up during formal class time.

During most of the sessions (always including the first) a couple from a previous series returns to tell their birth story. This presentation usually stimulates a lively discussion that brings home to the people in the class that they, too, will be giving birth soon.

The round robin is repeated at the start of every session. This time is used to elicit reactions to the previous class and to air any issues that have come up during the week.

Relaxation exercises early in the evening help lessen tension.

The discussion is geared to group interests, even if there is some deviation from the planned outline. Emotions should be allowed to surface and play themselves out. Moreover, group identity is strengthened by supporting individual members in crisis, with emotional release and physical contact encouraged. If interest in an issue lags, the leader should terminate the discussion and summarize areas of agreement.

Group consensus and the sensitivity of the instructor are relied on to determine when an individual life crisis (e.g., death of a parent) or obstetric problem (e.g., breech presentation) is relevant to the purposes of the group, and when a self-centered or chronically anxious person must be tactfully prevented from disrupting or monopolizing a session. The instructor should be prepared to deal with numerous ways in which the needs of a particular woman or couple may run counter to those of the group. Experienced parents should be reminded at the outset to be considerate of the needs of first-timers. People who have rigid expectations and are not receptive to the philosophy of the group should be given an opportunity to explore an alternative model in the form of a structured, hospital-based class such as Lamaze. Those who are shy should be drawn out. The leaders should sit next to very vocal participants to restrain them from monopolizing her attention. Overly optimistic people, who can undermine the seriousness of the group, need to be reminded continually that there are many kinds of birth experience. People who are very negative or critical need tactful acknowledgment, some time to talk, and then a firm cutoff coupled with an offer to talk outside the class. People with extreme fears or physical or emotional problems should be counseled to seek additional support from their midwife or physician or other personal counselor.

Participants are given a list of the class members with addresses, telephone numbers, and due dates and are encouraged to contact one another.

Facilitating Critical Discussion

A childbirth class should also serve as a milieu where people can critically evaluate their expectations and preconceived notions about birth, as well as those of their families and society. Although the instructor is herself committed to alternative birth practices, her role is not to proselytize for home birth from a strong ideological position but to open up questions for reexamination.

The instructor should stimulate discussion of issues such as the following:

- *family relationships*. Home birth adds fuel to the fire of family conflicts resulting from clashes of opinions and traditions.
- *pain and fear*. Couples should be encouraged to come to terms with all the sensations associated with birth: noise, mess, pain, fear, the sight and feel of blood. Discussion of these sensations, preceded and followed by a visualization exercise, can make them seem less alien and frightening. This discussion can begin with the question, "What did your mother tell you about birth?"

- *lack of predictability and control.* Many people are attached to the goal of controlling the events and sensations of birth. The great variation in normal births, plus examples of complications, are illustrated by couples who return to tell their birth stories.

- *risk and responsibility.* Areas covered include why people make the choices they do, who is responsible for which aspects of the birth, and what are the risks of home birth. Here, too, birth stories stimulate discussion.

- *death and injury.* The leader should introduce this topic if it does not arise spontaneously. Acknowledging even the most extreme fears during pregnancy is essential to realistic preparation for childbirth. (See discussion of pregnancy loss in Chapter 12.) Concrete examples of death or damage should be mentioned. People should not assume that it will not happen to them. On the other hand, dwelling on the negative too heavily can frighten people deeply and make them lose faith in themselves.

- *circumcision.* This is often a very controversial topic, which touches on other aspects of medical and personal decision making in pregnancy, such as risk and safety, family relationships (e.g., with prospective grandparents who have strong feelings on the matter), and the responsibility of making choices that the child must live with. Source materials on this and other subjects unrelated to home birth, which nonetheless entail difficult choices (e.g., amniocentesis[7]), should be made available.

The discussions in class should stimulate participants to explore their feelings on their own as individuals and couples. The instructor may wish to share the birth preference letters written by other couples. These documents can help families clarify their values and communicate their wishes to professional caregivers and institutions.

The instructor should encourage families to let go of expectations and to be prepared for a wide range of possible outcomes. The discussion of each issue should be summarized in positive but realistic terms.

Nurturing Positive Attitudes

Birth should be viewed not as a medical crisis but as a normal physiological process that a healthy woman's body can deal with. Throughout the class series the instructor can advocate, without imposing, attitudes about birth that are consistent with this view: namely, that labor is normal, healthy, and necessary for mother and baby; that a woman has unanticipated strength to deal with her labor; that her friends and attendants are there to help her tap this strength; that her body works and has a wisdom of its own; and that after the birth she will be able to mother and nurse her baby and take care of whatever she must attend to.

Emphasizing Normal Birth

Instruction should be kept simple and basic. Although complications of labor must be covered, they should not be given disproportionate emphasis.

An Eclectic Approach to Labor Support

Couples should be assisted in dealing with their pain and fear by the provision of a practical repertoire of labor supports, with emphasis on the family's capacity to discover what works for them. Although no one method is taught, people learn that there is much that can be done to help themselves have a baby easily and smoothly. Acquisition of skills to meet various contingencies itself allays fear.

Contact with Birth Attendants

Home birth educators and health care providers who have clients in common should establish channels of communication for dealing with clinical, logistical, political, and philosophical issues. Such contact may be difficult to achieve in areas where home birth education groups are in direct conflict with accepted obstetrical practices. Nonetheless, it is helpful to be able to exchange relevant information without breaching the confidentiality of either the attendant's or the educator's relationships with clients or compromising the role of the home birth education group as a milieu allowing for critical examination and discussion, one independent of any other organization or institution.

If, for example, a woman expresses dissatisfaction with a birth attendant or reveals a potentially serious inadequacy in her own preparation for birth, the educator should suggest strongly that she discuss it with the attendant. If on subsequent inquiry the client indicates that she has not done so, the educator may (when warranted) approach the attendant and say, "Did [the client] discuss [the problem] with you? I have a feeling that it's a serious issue for her." The educator should, however, be careful not to give the relationship with the attendant priority over the relationship with the woman or couple.

CLASS OUTLINE

The outline of the Birth Day classes presented in Exhibit 8-1 is an example of the organization and presentation of a childbirth education series. Classes are held one evening a week, each session lasting two and one-half to three hours. Couples may begin the series at any time during the pregnancy.

Recommended readings in each category can be selected from those listed in Appendix C. Rahima Baldwin's *Special Delivery*[8] is recommended as an overall resource book for the series. As new information becomes available it is incorporated into the classes.

Major Content Areas

This section deals with the content of the more important areas of teaching both for the class leader and the birth attendant. Although some topics are treated in greater depth than others, the reader should refer to other sources, including the other chapters of this book cross-referenced here, for additional information on all the subjects listed. The International Childbirth Education Association's Bookcenter offers a complete selection of further reading (see Appendix B).

Nutrition

Nutrition is the factor over which the pregnant woman has the most influence and is probably at least as important in determining the outcome of her pregnancy as her health care. Fortunately, most potential clients of a home birth practice are already aware of these facts even before pregnancy. For those who are not, classes, books, and the advice of the attendant are usually convincing.

Childbirth educators may choose to include nutrition evaluation in their classes in the form of either individual or group self-evaluation. In any case, childbirth classes should reinforce the evaluation and counseling by the attendant (see Chapter 7). Families and instructors can share appealing recipes or other nutritional suggestions. They should also be encouraged to discuss unusual or controversial nutritional philosophies. The primary aim, however, is to instill the idea that good nutrition is vital. This notion is reinforced when couples who have given birth describe to the expectant couples that their beautiful, healthy babies are products of well-nourished pregnancies.

Exhibit 8-1 Outline of Birth Day Classes

Class I
- A. Introductions
- B. Discussion of individual expectations about pregnancy and birth
- C. Relaxation exercise
- D. Presentation by couple who have had a home birth
- E. Recommended readings for Class II on exercise, nutrition, drugs in pregnancy, and fetal growth and development

Class II
- A. Continuation of relaxation
- B. Anatomy and physiology of pregnancy
- C. Prenatal exercises
- D. Nutrition for pregnancy, birth and lactation
- E. Preparation of nipples for breast-feeding
- F. Recommended readings for Class III on labor and birth

Class III
- A. Relaxation and birth visualization
- B. Physiology of labor and birth
- C. Introduction of labor supports
- D. Recommended readings for Classes IV and V on options in childbirth and emergency procedures

Class IV
- A. Touch relaxation
- B. Positions for labor and birth
- C. Labor supports (continued)
- D. Birthing room couple

Class V
- A. Touch relaxation
- B. Preparation of home/birth room, friends and siblings
- C. Tapes of births
- D. Emotional and psychological issues of labor and birth
- E. Recommended readings for Class VI on cesarean sections and other complications

Class VI
- A. Establishing your birthing priorities
- B. Possible complications and medical emergencies
- C. Hospital preparation
- D. Discussion of individual concerns and expectations
- E. Recommended readings for Classes VII and VIII on breast-feeding and postpartum and newborn care

Class VII
- A. Anticipating the newborn
- B. Discussion of effects and possible complications of routine vitamin K, eye prophylaxis, circumcision. On what basis do we, as parents, make decisions for our baby?
- C. Breast-feeding
- D. Movie of home birth

Exhibit 8-1 continued

Class VIII
  A. Emotional and practical issues for parents in the postpartum period
  B. What to expect as the baby grows
  C. Postpartum couple
  D. Recommended readings on parenting, breast-feeding, and family planning to keep at hand as the baby grows

Responsibility

Responsibility is a central theme of home birth. Although responsible adulthood cannot be taught, how to act responsibly in a given situation can be modeled.[9] At the same time, the emphasis on participatory effort in home birth should not be allowed to obscure the element of uncertainty involved in the outcome. As important as it is to eat well, exercise, take part in the classes, avoid harmful drugs, wear seat belts in automobiles, and so forth, these precautions do not guarantee an uncomplicated birth and a healthy baby; they merely improve the odds. Responsibility, then, should not mean guilt in the event of a bad outcome.

Childbirth classes should play a part in educating people to be responsible. They should be a forum for the discussion of risks, benefits, responsibilities, and values involved in making choices. Home birth is much more than a choice of a type of service. It is a choice of an attitude, a stance, and a willingness to bring elemental forces into one's private domain. Although the risks of home birth are not necessarily greater than those of hospital birth, they have a different character. Practical yet life-and-death decisions may arise, not all of which would present themselves in the hospital. For example, if the mother has had postpartum hemorrhage that is brought under control, she and her male partner will need to decide whether he can be comfortable taking care of her or whether she should be transferred to the hospital for further surveillance. They must also come to terms with how the choice of home birth will influence society's view of the outcome. If parents do not understand the full extent of these responsibilities, they cannot know whether or not they are prepared to assume them.

Family-Centered Birth with Sibling Preparation and Participation

Childbirth education should take into account the needs of the family as a whole, including the prospective father, siblings, grandparents, aunts, and uncles. In addition, a home birth often directly involves friends as well as relatives. Preparation of siblings for birth deserves special mention.

Before the birth there are various projects that can help prepare a child for the new baby. Examples include dyeing T-shirts for the whole family (including the new baby) to be worn at the birth, making a quilt, soft toys, or mobiles, or making special food to be eaten at the birth. Parents can be encouraged to be original and inventive and to contribute their ideas to others. Projects should be pleasurable while permitting the child to participate with other family members in planning for the baby. In conjunction with these projects, clear and appropriate explanations and answers to questions can be given to the child about the "mechanics" of pregnancy and birth. Parents should be alert for and should correct children's distorted views of birth. Verbal descriptions can be supplemented by books, pictures, and sounds (either taped or imitated); visits to the physician, midwife, childbirth education class, or hospital; and participation in the mother's exercises. Material used will depend on the age and temperament of the child.

During birth it is important to use recognizable words, similar to those used in preparation, to describe what is happening. One person previously identified to the child is designated as the child's caretaker. This person is at the birth primarily to care for the child: to answer questions, feed and nurture the child, and leave the room if the child does. The child should be told ahead of time that it is likely that neither mommy nor daddy will be able to take care of him or her during the birth. If the parents are comfortable having the child in the room where labor and delivery take place, the child should be free to choose whether or not to be in that room. The caretaker understands that he or she may miss the birth if the child decides not to be present.

After the birth it is very important not to forget the older child while lost in the wonder of the newborn. Time spent with the sibling as soon as possible after the birth will help ease tensions and jealousies later on. Reading or telling stories, presenting a new toy, and simply being with the child are activities that can go on while the baby is sleeping or is with someone else.

Parents expecting a second child often worry about how the family's needs may change and about how to approach the older child. These issues can be addressed in childbirth classes. Together with the questions of sibling preparation and participation discussed above, they are also covered in greater detail in a booklet entitled "Children at Birth," by Jenifer M. Fleming, which can be obtained from Birth Day (see Appendix B).

Exercise and Relaxation (see Chapter 9)

Labor Support

Labor support in the home can be much more varied and can be shared with many more people than in the hospital. Prenatal teaching should attempt to instill a sense of flexibility and creativity and deemphasize rigid breathing techniques (see Chapter 11).

Physiology of Birth and Birth Procedures

Physiology of birth and birth procedures should be discussed so that parents can evaluate different techniques. The importance of finding out the attendant's preferences regarding birth position (if charts are used, hold them so that the birth is not always shown in a supine position), criteria for episiotomy, use of prophylactic eye medication or vitamin K, and length of the third stage that is considered normal should be stressed. Even if the attendant has no set practices, it is useful to try to give the family a picture of how an attendant might be expected to handle the events of birth.

Complications of Labor and Birth

Common complications of labor and birth, as outlined in Chapter 11, must be discussed as a matter of routine, with emphasis on newborn resuscitation and maternal hemorrhage. If the parents want to know more or if the attendant or instructor believes that the parents need to be more realistic, other complications should be dealt with as well.

Newborn Care (see Chapter 12)

Postpartum Care (see Chapter 13)

Breast-feeding

Breast-feeding is particularly important after a home birth (to ensure involution of the uterus and to avoid the potential complications of initiating formula feeding). Preparation for breast-feeding, physiological functioning of the breasts, and the art of breast-feeding itself should be covered. La Leche League and Nursing Mothers' Council both welcome pregnant women to their meetings. Health Education Associates has an excellent handout on prenatal breast preparation (see Appendices A and B for addresses).

THE POSTPARTUM CLASS

On the night of the last prenatal class a postpartum class is scheduled for a date after every participant's due date. Scheduling a postpartum group in advance gives people a reason to keep in touch with other class members after their babies are born and to bring people together again around parenting issues. Building this idea into the class series fosters support and trading of services, pot lucks, and gatherings after the births. Many groups of "alumni" of Birth Day series still meet in one another's homes.

USE OF BOOKS AND VISUALS IN HOME BIRTH EDUCATION

In Birth Day instructional materials are kept simple. The physiology of pregnancy and the development of the fetus are illustrated by five plates from the Maternity Center Association in New York, while the physiology of labor and birth is depicted in five plates from Midwest ParentCraft Center in Illinois (see Appendices A and B for addresses). In using the latter it is a good idea to lead a visualization exercise a week before introducing the plates so that each participant can imagine the changes her cervix will undergo during labor before seeing a full-color likeness.

Essential to any home birth education class is an up-to-date library with a wide range of books on birth, pregnancy, breast-feeding, and postpartum issues, representing different philosophies and points of view. Even so, information has its costs as well as benefits. A good teacher respects individual learning styles. In addition to color plates, therefore, slides, drawings, audiotapes, and films are used. One of the best teaching tools of all is a couple relating their birth experience before the class.

CONCLUSION

Childbirth education, like childbirth, involves a considerable amount of detail. To keep the larger issues in perspective, these words by Sheila Kitzinger are relevant:

> Childbirth Education is not so much a matter of teaching exercises, instructing a coach in how to use a stopwatch, introducing new techniques of management into obstetrics and getting flowered drapes hung in the delivery room, as it is in helping each person, and each couple realize their own potential for creative experience as they give birth to their babies.[10]

Childbirth education as envisioned in this chapter and as practiced in Birth Day and similar groups is not primarily about anatomy and physiology but about people. The childbirth educator, like the birth attendant, has an opportunity and a responsibility to engage with people in their wholeness, individuality, and common humanity.

NOTES

1. Louise Trusler Mangan and Karen E. May, "Conference Report: Midwifery is . . . A Labour of Love," *Women and Health* 5, no. 2 (Summer 1980): 102–104.

2. Harold Bursztajn et al., *Medical Choices, Medical Chances: How Patients, Families, and Physicians Can Cope With Uncertainty* (New York: Delacorte Press/Seymour Lawrence, 1981), pp. 349–388.

3. Sheila Kitzinger, *Education and Counseling for Childbirth* (New York: Schocken, 1979), p. 40.

4. Michel Odent, Lecture presented at Boston University, Boston, Massachusetts, 1980.

5. Anne S. Kasper, "Independent Practice as a Nurse-Midwife in Bethesda, Maryland: An Interview with Jan Epstein, CNM," *Women and Health* 6, no. 4 (Winter 1981): 181.

6. Mary Howell, *Healing at Home: A Guide to Health Care for Children* (Boston: Beacon Press, 1979).

7. Susan Perlmutter Pauker and Stephen G. Pauker, "The Amniocentesis Decision: An Explicit Guide for Parents," *Birth Defects: Original Article Series* 15 (1979): 289–324.

8. Rahima Baldwin, *Special Delivery* (Millbrae, Calif.: Les Femmes Publishing, 1979).

9. Doris Haire et al., *The Pregnant Patient's Bill of Rights, The Pregnant Patient's Responsibilities* (Minneapolis: International Childbirth Education Association, 1977).

10. Kitzinger, *Education and Counseling for Childbirth*, p. ix.

Chapter 9

Prenatal Exercise

Elizabeth Noble, R.P.T.

With improvements in maternity care, the focus of childbirth education in recent years has been expanded beyond preparation for labor and delivery to encompass a broad range of issues in the childbearing year, including prenatal and postpartum exercise, physical fitness, and an understanding of body mechanics.

The purpose of prenatal exercise is not only to improve muscle strength, but also, and equally important, to stretch tight muscles. Muscles are tense and shortened as often as they are weak. Improvement of the musculoskeletal system through a balanced program of exercise and relaxation helps to prevent or alleviate many common discomforts of pregnancy, such as backache, varicose veins, cramps, constipation, breathlessness, heartburn, and postural discomfort. A woman in good physical condition will be better able to withstand the rigors of a long or difficult labor. Such condition takes time to develop.

Prenatal exercise also has indirect benefits that enhance the birth experience. Women who exercise regularly throughout pregnancy gain heightened body awareness, confidence in their physiological functions, and knowledge of how these are affected by the changes brought on by pregnancy. Exercise skills are less easily learned by women who present in the third trimester for childbirth preparation. A woman who learns to "bond with her body" can better trust her uterus and "let go" during labor. Clearly, the sooner a pregnant woman begins exercising, the better.

CHOOSING AN EXERCISE CLASS

Exercise classes for pregnant women provide interaction with other expectant mothers. The classes may be separate from or part of the general childbirth education classes for childbearing couples described in the previous chapter. Much general information can be imparted informally during exercise classes.

Although there are increasing numbers of obstetric-gynecologic physical therapists who are trained to provide the best musculoskeletal care during the childbearing year, in many communities there are no classes at all. Health spas, fitness centers, or dance schools may offer prenatal or postpartum exercises, with great variation in quality. However, as long as a woman listens to her body and does nothing that causes strain or pain, then she can usually reap the benefits and avoid the hazards.

Unfortunately, many of these exercise programs neglect the pelvic floor and reflect little understanding of physiological changes in pregnancy. The ideal exercise class has a small number of participants who are individually evaluated and supervised rather than trained to "follow the leader" in strenuous activities. The rationale for each position and movement should be explained, along with the role of the muscles in pregnancy, birth, and post partum. Exercises are best presented in a broad context, coordinated with breathing, relaxation, and preparation for birth.

ESSENTIAL EXERCISES FOR THE CHILDBEARING YEAR

A suggested exercise program lasts for one and one-half hours and is divided into sessions of calisthenics, stretching, and relaxation. Exercises need be done only a few times to be beneficial but must be performed slowly and properly. Jerking and straining must be avoided. The goal is increased body awareness and comfort, not training for the Olympics. Quivering of muscles or the use of sudden jerky movements designed to bypass a weak muscle group indicates that the exercise is too difficult and should be modified. Once an exercise is mastered and is no longer taxing, it is preferable to make the exercise more challenging by changing the leverage of the body and the effect of gravity rather than merely to increase the number of repetitions. Much re-education is also required to convince the average person that an exercise is worthwhile even if it does not hurt.

Breathing must at all times be coordinated with exercise movements. An easy guideline is "Exhale during exertion." This avoids the adverse cardiovascular effects of the Valsalva maneuver (effort against a closed glottis). Furthermore, venous return is actually improved as positive pressure is maintained in the abdomen and negative pressure in the thorax.

The woman should become aware of and harmonize her movement with the natural expansion of the chest and abdomen during inspiration and with their relaxation during exhalation. This may need supervision initially, since reverse diaphragmatic breathing is not uncommon. Abdominal tightening on outward breath is a good preliminary exercise and demonstrates the role of the abdominal muscles in forced exhalation.

The following exercises, illustrated in Figure 9-1, are condensed from *Essential Exercises for the Childbearing Year* by Elizabeth Noble.[1] Exercise programs can, of course, be expanded beyond the basic principles and movements outlined here. However, it is important that the muscles

---

Figure 9-1 Summary of Essential Prenatal Exercises

Do each exercise twice at first, progressing at your own pace to 5 times. The sequence can be repeated in reverse order. Relax and breathe deeply between each exercise.

1. Deep breathing with Abdominal-Wall–Tightening on outward breath

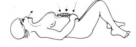

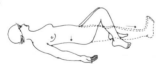

2. Foot Exercises: stretch, bend, and rotate

3. Stretch out the Kinks: on the bed, against wall

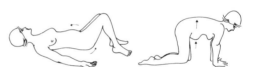

4. Pelvic Floor: 4 exercises

5. Pelvic-Tilting: various positions

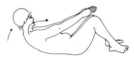

6. Leg-Sliding

7. Straight Curl-up

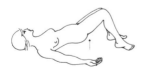

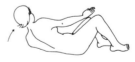

8. Bridging

9. Diagonal Curl-up

When *standing up*, roll over onto the knees and push arm with the arms. When rising from the floor, go on to one knee and straighten legs to stand (page 106).

10. *Posture Check:* (page 161).

Relaxation session: Twenty minutes' complete tension release in any position of comfort twice daily.

Source: Reprinted from *Essential Exercises for the Childbearing Year,* 2nd ed. rev., by Elizabeth Noble, with permission of Houghton Mifflin Company, © 1982.

stressed most by childbearing—the abdominals and the pelvic floor—receive the most emphasis. Both are weak in the average person. In general, women have poor awareness of the pelvic floor. While more visible, the abdominal muscles are rarely exercised in a society in which people mostly sit or stand. In pregnancy these muscles must meet the demands of increased weight gain, changes in the center of gravity, and support for the enlarging uterus.

Abdominal and Back Muscle Exercises

It is usually not appreciated that the abdominal wall muscles provide much of the support for the spine and therefore play an important role in the health of the back. Together with the gluteus maximus muscles, the abdominals control the angle of the pelvis in relation to the spine, an angle that affects stability and stress of the lower back. A common view is that backache is due to a weakness of the back muscles. However, these muscles are usually, if anything, too tight rather than too weak. Thus, the abdominals are emphasized in back conditioning programs.

During pregnancy the axis of contraction between the origin and insertion of the abdominals changes from a straight line between the pelvis and ribs to an increasing curve between these upper and lower attachments as the abdominal wall stretches to accommodate the uterus. Therefore, it makes sense to embark on abdominal strengthening exercises as early as possible. The abdominal muscles are exercised by two main movements against gravity: trunk curl-ups with the pelvis stabilized and pelvic tilting combined with leg lowering while the trunk is stabilized. The knees are flexed, and the lower back is never allowed to arch (i.e., the posterior pelvic tilt is maintained at all times). Thus, there is no threat of injury to the lumbar area during any of the following exercises.

Curl-ups: Regular and Modified

Curl-ups finish short of contraction of the hip flexors (iliopsoas), and therefore the trunk is never brought forward more than 45 degrees, for some people much less. The waist always stays on the floor. In order to exercise all components of the abdominal musculature, curl-ups are done in both straight and diagonal directions. During the diagonal curl-up each shoulder is turned toward the opposite knee. The effort of the abdominals can be increased progressively by changing the position of the arms:

- In the initial position, the arms reach toward the knees, assisting the movement (60 percent abdominal muscle effort).

- The next progression involves a neutral position with arms folded across the chest (80 percent effort).
- Finally, the arms are clasped behind the head to increase the leverage (100 percent effort).

Each woman must begin at the appropriate entry level and progress at her own pace. Obviously, the physical changes that occur in later pregnancy may make advanced curl-ups too difficult.

Diastasis Recti. It is important to check for any separation of the recti abdominus muscles at the linea alba (diastasis recti). This condition is usually observed after the fifth month but may be seen earlier in multiparae whose diastases have remained since the previous pregnancy (Figure 9-2). Many women notice the bulging in the midline of the abdominal wall

---

Figure 9-2 Diastasis Recti

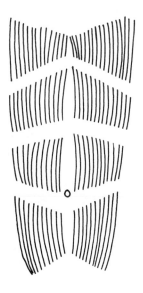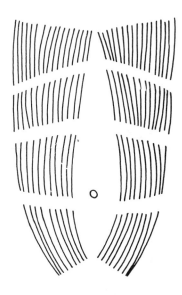

The recti muscles can separate as a zipper opens under stress.

Source: Reprinted from *Essential Exercises for the Childbearing Year,* 2nd ed. rev., by Elizabeth Noble, with permission of Houghton Mifflin Company, © 1982.

during exercises, as they get up off the floor afterward, or as they get out of bed or the bath. Diastasis recti is quite painless, but it may lead to postural backache secondary to abdominal wall weakness. Factors that predispose to this condition include hormonal softening of myofascial structures, decreased general tonus and condition of the muscular system, persistent straining (as with chronic constipation or obstructive pulmonary disease), harmful exercises (e.g., full sit-ups with extended legs and double-leg raising), hereditary tendencies, and abdominal surgery.

To check for diastasis recti, the woman lies supine with the knees flexed. She raises her head (which activates the recti muscles), allowing her hands to reach toward her knees. The woman or the attendant notes any herniation present. It is always possible to palpate with one or two fingers between the recti. However, if three or more fingers can be placed between the contracted recti muscles, then the diagnosis of diastasis recti is made.

A woman with a diastasis should avoid strong fixation work required of the abdominal wall as in curl-ups, double-leg lowering exercises (to be described later), and any heavy lifting or straining. She should also take care when arising from the floor to roll over and push herself into a sitting position with her arms. Couples can be reassured that it is easy to "close the gap" with exercises post partum, but improvement cannot be expected in pregnancy as there will be continued stretching of the abdominal wall. Women with diastasis recti do not usually have difficulty with second stage of labor since the uterus normally performs most of the expulsive effort.

The diagnosis of diastasis recti requires that a woman's exercise program be modified with regard to curl-ups. To perform the modified curl-up (Figure 9-3), the woman with a diastasis recti lies supine with knees flexed and hands crossed at the area of the gap to support the recti muscles. Head raises only are performed, taking care that the abdominal wall is pulled in as the breath is exhaled, so as not to increase the bulging. The emphasis is on doing the exercises frequently.

The same program is followed post partum, after a check for a diastasis on about the third day. After a few days post partum the woman can evaluate the gap when performing the exercise without hand support. If the muscles are parallel at the midline, she can then slowly progress by bringing the shoulders off the horizontal, but only little by little. Too rapid progression can lead to reseparation.

Avoid Sit-ups. A difference must be noted between curl-ups and the kind of sit-ups that unfortunately remain popular in many fitness classes. First, with curl-ups the knees are flexed to stabilize the lumbar spine and decrease the effect of the hip flexors. The movement also is limited to the abdominals and is never more than 45 degrees forward flexion. A sit-up, which pri-

Figure 9-3 Modified Curl-Up for Women with Diastasis Recti

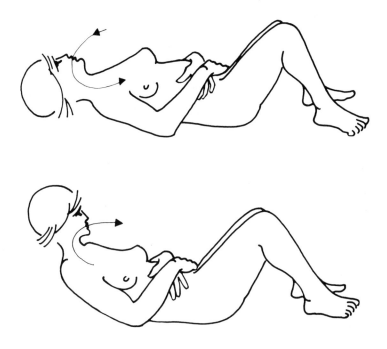

Support the recti muscles as you raise your head on outward breath.

Source: Reprinted from *Essential Exercises for the Childbearing Year,* 2nd ed. rev., by Elizabeth Noble, with permission of Houghton Mifflin Company, © 1982.

marily involves a 90-degree movement, is actually performed primarily by the iliopsoas, which pulls the lumbar spine into a lordosis. The abdominals, on the other hand, roll the body forward, as the ribs approach the pelvis and there is no strain on the lumbar spine. The second half of the sit-up hardly exercises the abdominals at all and may actually conceal weak abdominal muscles, as is typically seen in the person who jerks quickly through the first phase of the movement. Extending the legs and fixing the feet with external force further encourages action of the iliopsoas and increases the lumbar strain.

Pelvic Tilting and Bridging

Pelvic-tilting movements focus on the lower part of the abdominal wall and can be done in many positions. The action is to flatten the curve of the lower spine by squeezing the buttocks tightly together and pulling in the abdominals, tilting the pelvis posteriorly. In the correct position the anterior-superior iliac spine and the pubic symphysis are aligned in the same frontal plane.

Like curl-ups, pelvic tilting exercises can be done progressively in three different positions while supine. In contrast to curl-ups the legs rather than the arms are adjusted. The knees are flexed, and the feet are flat on the floor. With heels sliding along the floor the legs are extended as far as possible while the pelvic tilt is maintained. Eventually the tilt will be possible with the legs fully extended. Finally, with the tilt maintained the legs and thighs are raised to a vertical position with the knees bent. Then the thighs and legs are simultaneously and gradually lowered and extended to the point where the pelvic tilt is maximally stressed yet maintained. Usually the point is reached before 45 degrees of leg lowering has occurred (100 percent lower abdominal strength). Many women will be able to lower the legs to 45 degrees only after considerable practice.

Avoid Double-Leg Raising. The significant difference between double-leg raising and leg lowering as described is that in the latter the individual is in control of the lowering movement at all times. That is, the legs are not lowered or straightened beyond the point of the abdominal muscles' ability to maintain the lumbar area flat on the floor. Therefore, no harm results. The problem with double-leg raising is that during the most difficult initial part of the movement the pelvic tilt is out of control because the iliopsoas dominates, not the abdominals. As with a seesaw, the short lever of the pelvis rises before the longer lever of the outstretched legs. This exercise has caused much discomfort and worsening of back pain. Anybody can raise or lower the legs. The point is to be able to maintain the pelvic tilt and protect the lumbar spine while the muscles that do so are stressed and thereby strengthened. Double-leg raising should be eliminated from any exercise program, especially those designed for childbearing women.

Basic pelvic tilting can also be done in sitting, standing, kneeling, side-lying, and all-fours positions. There are progressive exercises for the all-fours position, but supervision is required, since many errors can occur. While maintaining a pelvic tilt (keeping the back and pelvis "as flat as a tabletop"), first one arm at a time, then one leg at a time is extended. The final progression is to extend contralateral arm and leg together. In this exercise the abdominals and gluteals hold the pelvis in line with the spine against gravity and the changing leverage of different arm and leg positions. The all-fours position relieves backache and pressure from the uterus, and the progressive exercises improve balance and strengthen the arms. This is a good substitute for the woman with a diastasis who cannot do curl-ups.

Bridging is the act of raising the buttocks off the floor while lying supine. It helps improve the pelvic tilt by strengthening the gluteal muscles, which pull the pelvis down in conjunction with the upward movement of the abdominals. As these muscles are unaffected by the growing uterus, the pregnant woman may have more awareness of their contraction than that of the abdominals. Bridging is preferably done with the legs extended and heels resting on a low table or footstool. The buttocks are lifted from the floor to form a bridge with the body. If this exercise is done with the knees bent, the woman must be taught to feel the difference between gluteal contractions and the leverage exerted by the hamstrings. The farther the heels are from the buttocks, the less substitution occurs with the hamstrings, which can extend the hips when the knees are bent. Bridging should be done with the pelvic tilt in place and buttocks held as firm as possible.

Pelvic Floor Exercises

The importance of various musculofascial layers that comprise the pelvic floor, particularly the pubococcygeus, cannot be overemphasized. They are typically neglected. The three main functions of the pelvic floor are (1) support of the pelvic organs, viscera, and the increasing weight of the uterus in pregnancy; (2) sphincteric control of the anus and urethra; and (3) sexual response, which is enhanced by healthy muscles that can provide proprioceptive stimulation during intercourse, adequate orgasmic platform, and reflex muscular contractions during orgasm.

Structural changes in the pelvic floor, such as laxity, various degrees of uterine prolapse, cystocele, rectocele, and enterocele affect many women in Western society.[2] Functional changes, such as urinary stress incontinence, lack of sexual satisfaction for either partner, and incomplete elimination are also very common. Most women believe that stress incontinence and "falling-out feelings" are a normal side effect of pregnancy, since many of their friends suffer the same symptoms. Smoking, obesity, and chronic chest conditions, which cause increases in intraabdominal pressure, all aggravate pelvic floor dysfunction. Although hormonal softening and some descent of the pelvic floor are physiological during pregnancy, adequate urinary control can and should be maintained throughout.

Healthy pelvic floor tissues can facilitate safe progress through the second stage of labor. A well-exercised vascular muscle can better withstand distention before its fibers become anoxic or torn. As Dr. Arnold Kegel shows in his film on pelvic floor dynamics, a strong muscle remains protected by the pubic rami during crowning, whereas a thin, fibrous pubococcygeus is dragged down with the fetal head and is more likely to be injured.[3] Also important for preserving an intact perineum is the conduct of the second stage of labor, as described in Chapter 11.

There are many difficulties in learning to contract the pubococcygeus, a movement in which no bones move, the action being internal and out of sight. Without some sort of biofeedback, women may be only minimally aware of their efforts and hence discouraged. Many have problems identifying the pubococcygeus and cannot contract it in isolation from other muscle groups. Typically, accessory muscles such as the adductors, glutei, and abdominals are substituted (which along with breath-holding results in a bearing-down action rather than an uplifting contraction of the pelvic floor). Since vaginal examinations are not performed during exercise or childbirth classes, it is essential that the attendant verify the location and correct action of the pubococcygeus for the woman, perhaps with the aid of illustrations, if she cannot do so herself.

Once a woman has identified the correct muscle, she tightens the anal and vaginal sphincters, thereby also raising the perineum. The rising of an elevator and drawing up of a hammock are helpful analogies. Muscular contractions must be done slowly enough to recruit as many muscle fibers as possible. Contract/relax exercises (also known as "kegeling") can be done at any time. In particular, the pelvic floor should be braced during exertion such as sneezing, coughing, or lifting. A useful test for the woman is to interrupt her urine flow. Those who cannot do this will need special re-education of the muscle. To facilitate contraction, the attendant can elicit the stretch reflex by digitally stretching the vagina while the woman simultaneously squeezes. In some cases, treatment with a biofeedback device under the supervision of a physical therapist may be required. Kegel's perineometer at one time was used but is no longer available. A newly developed device, the "electronic perineometer" (available from a firm listed in Appendix B), measures the microvoltage of the pubococcygeus and uses auditory and visual biofeedback with standard electromyographic apparatus. This instrument not only improves muscle strength but also assists in the release of chronic pelvic floor tension, which may be associated with chronic vaginal infection or prolonged second stage.

Research has shown that the pelvic floor readily fatigues with exercise and that the average person cannot do more than a few contractions of consistent strength.[4] Similarly, holding a contraction for more than 10 seconds is beyond the ability of most nonconditioned women. Instructions should state clearly that the exercises should be done "little and often," just three or four in a series followed by a rest interval. A total of about 50 should be done daily. Sexual intercourse is another obvious opportunity for the practice and improvement of pelvic floor control, with the added advantage of partner feedback. Pelvic floor exercises can be done anywhere at any time. They should become as routine as brushing the teeth.

Stretching Exercises

Flexibility is as important as strength for health and well-being. The muscle groups that typically are tight are the hamstrings, calf muscles, hip flexors, and back extensors. The easiest general stretch is to lie supine and press the spinal curves as much as possible into the floor. The hamstrings can be stretched by standing with one leg elevated on a chair or table, or by long sitting (legs outstretched) or lying supine and elevating one straight leg at a time. In pregnancy these positions are preferable to bending forward, which usually involves rounding of the back and excess pressure on vertebral disks. It is important to flex the hips rather than the spine, since the hamstrings are attached to the ischial tuberosities. Calf-stretching can be done half-kneeling with the foot of the forward leg firmly applied to the floor as weight is shifted progressively forward or standing with one foot in front of the other with the knee of the rear leg kept extended and the foot planted on the floor as the front knee is flexed. The hip flexors can also be stretched in the half-kneeling position, one foot in front and the other leg extended behind, with the weight transferred onto the forward foot until a stretch is felt in the opposite groin. The back can be stretched in tailor-sitting position (hips abducted, knees bent) with trunk flexion bringing the head toward the floor and half tailor-sitting with trunk flexion to either side. Sitting with the legs extended (long sit) and holding the back at a 90-degree angle or bending further at the waist is an excellent stretch and postural exercise. The back extensors can be worked by pressing the spine against a wall, and the exercise can be made more difficult by abducting and elevating the arms while maintaining contact with the wall. Squatting is another recommended stretching position, which can be a useful position for second stage. Those with tight heel cords need to begin with shoes on until the heels can rest on the floor without pronation of the feet. The abductors can be stretched in a sitting position with the soles of the feet together, allowing the force of gravity to abduct the thighs further. The "pelvic clock" exercise of Moshe Feldenkrais[5] can also be done in this position. This maneuver involves sitting in a chair with the soles of feet together and rotating the pelvis in a circle, first in one direction and then in the other. It is recommended for increasing pelvic awareness. Other stretching exercises can be found in *Stretching* by Bob Anderson[6] and the *Runner's World Yoga Book* by Jean Couch and Nell Weaver.[7] These simple guides, suitable for beginners, emphasize the point that stretching must be slow, static, and sustained. Bouncing must always be avoided because it activates the neuromuscular stretch reflex.

Women should be encouraged to continue with their favorite sports and to listen to their bodies for signs about how much to do as the pregnancy progresses. Many expectant mothers take yoga classes or belly dancing, which are most helpful in physical preparation and body awareness.

Aerobic Exercise

Aerobic exercise can be achieved by a combination of walking, skipping, jumping, jogging, and dancing, using backward, forward, and sideways directions for variety. The "warm-up" and "cool-down" must not be overlooked, and the woman should be taught how to count her heart rate. Other aerobic activities include jogging, cross-country skiing, brisk walking, and non-weight-bearing activities such as swimming, cycling, or exercises on large gymnastic balls.

Research in progress suggests that aerobic exercise in late pregnancy may not be entirely beneficial. Further clarification of this question is needed.

Relaxation

Relaxation must always receive emphasis in an exercise program. The ability to relax is a great asset for birth. The couple must learn that actively "being" is as important as "doing."

In fact, relaxation cannot be taught. People learn how to do it indirectly. Although childbirth classes often include training for "conscious release," physiologically this is not possible, since the receptors controlling muscle tension do not reach a conscious level in the brain. Messages are relayed to the cortex via proprioceptors. Thus the most effective "bodywork" approach is to work the antagonist to achieve relaxation of the agonist. Examples of this include "drag down the shoulders" for a tense and elevated shoulder girdle, "fingers long" to extend the overactive finger flexors, and "drag down the jaw" for tension in the face. Further details of this approach, which works on key areas of tension in the body, can be found in *Simple Relaxation* by Laura Mitchell.[8]

Mental relaxation must be encouraged along with physical release. These skills form the basis of yoga and meditation programs. Focusing on the natural rhythms of the breath will quiet the mind and facilitate general body relaxation. Controlling the breath requires effort, diminishes body awareness, and impairs relaxation. Couples can experience these phenomena for themselves by alternating observation and control of the breath.

The passive state of mental relaxation can also be obtained by silently repeating the number "one" as described in Herbert Benson's *The Relaxation Response*[9], by using a mantra as in meditation, or by guided fantasy and visualization.

CHANGING EMPHASIS IN PHYSICAL PREPARATION FOR CHILDBIRTH

As childbirth education comes of age, many of its practitioners are reevaluating traditional psychoprophylactic breathing techniques. Increasingly these are considered to be excessively rigid and nonphysiological (which in no way invalidates their historical importance in helping return control of childbearing to women). Even in home birth classes there is sometimes a preoccupation with rules of breathing rather than simply breathing spontaneously according to internal cues. Purposeful alteration of breathing with the goal of pain control consumes energy and limits feeling and awareness. Most couples who experience natural childbirth report that lack of energy is a more common difficulty during labor than unbearable pain. Much of the pain results from anxiety, tension, and fatigue that ironically may be exacerbated by the distraction techniques and breathing interventions taught by well-intentioned childbirth educators and birth attendants.

Shallow chest breathing has the disadvantage of not permitting sufficient air to traverse the anatomical dead space for adequate gaseous exchange to occur in the alveoli. On the other hand, if this type of breathing becomes rapid, hyperventilation symptoms may occur as the woman accelerates her breathing to "stay on top" of the intensifying contractions. Hyperventilation leads to respiratory alkalosis with vasoconstriction and changes in the oxyhemoglobin disassociation curve. As a result, flow is decreased and the blood can carry less oxygen. These changes could be significant if the fetus were depressed for any reason. More research on this question is needed.

Although women are commonly taught in classes to achieve an inverse relationship between depth and speed of respiration, research has shown that women in labor do not decrease their tidal volumes as the breathing rate increases.[10] Respiratory rate is the only practical guide for couples. It should not be more than 25 per minute, and ideally much less, to stay within physiological limits.

There is also growing awareness of the hazards of the Valsalva maneuver in the second stage during pushing. Traditionally, these forced expulsive efforts against a closed glottis have been taught in childbirth classes and enthusiastically encouraged by coaches. However, the closed pressure system that is formed leads to increased thoracic pressure, reduced venous return, and a fall in cardiac output. Repeated Valsalva maneuvers elevate the blood pressure, while prolonged Valsalva maneuvers result in low blood pressure. Use of the Valsalva maneuver in the second stage for more than five seconds leads to uteroplacental insufficiency and fetal hypoxia.[11] This is seen with type II dips in the fetal heart rate on the electronic fetal monitor (late deceleration and slow recovery).

Childbirth education should be kept simple, with emphasis on natural events and normal physiology, not on contrived techniques. If a couple and their attendants can learn to view childbirth as an involuntary process, one that need only be allowed to happen rather than controlled, the laboring woman will be better able to direct her energy within instead of dissipating it by attempting to put her mind outside her body. Women need to gain trust in their bodies, which is difficult with the extreme medicalization of health care, especially birth, that has occurred in our society. Exercise classes, begun early in pregnancy, are an excellent way to foster this self-reliance.

NOTES

1. Elizabeth Noble, *Essential Exercises for the Childbearing Year,* 2nd ed. rev. (Boston: Houghton Mifflin, 1982).

2. Robert Zacharin, "A Chinese Anatomy—The Pelvic Supporting Tissues of Chinese and Occidental Woman Compared and Contrasted," *Australian and New Zealand Journal of Obstetrics and Gynaecology* 17, no. 1 (February 1977): 28–32.

3. Arnold Kegel, *The Pathologic Condition of the Pubococcygeus Muscle in Women* (film) (Hollywood, Calif.: Morgan Camera Shop, 1953).

4. D. B. Scott et al., "Pelvic Faradism: Detailed Technique," *Physiotherapy* 57 (1971): 322–325.

5. Moshe Feldenkrais, *Awareness Through Movement* (New York: Harper & Row, 1972).

6. Bob Anderson, *Stretching* (Bolinas, Calif.: Shelter Publications, 1980).

7. Jean Couch with Nell Weaver, *The Runner's World Yoga Book* (Mountain View, Calif.: Anderson World, 1979).

8. Laura Mitchell, *Simple Relaxation: The Physiological Method for Easing Tension* (New York: Atheneum, 1979).

9. Herbert Benson, *The Relaxation Response* (New York: Morrow, 1975).

10. Joan McLaren, "Maternal Respiration in Labour." Paper presented at the World Confederation of Physical Therapy Convention, Tel Aviv, Israel, May 1978, based on research conducted by the Physiotherapy Department, Bristol Maternity Hospital, Bristol, England.

11. Roberto Caldeyro-Barcia, "The Influence of Maternal Bearing-Down Efforts in the Second Stage of Labor on Fetal Well-Being," in P. Simkin and C. Reinke, eds., *Kaleidoscope of Childbearing: Preparation, Birth and Nurturing* (Seattle: the pennypress, 1978), pp. 31–42.

Chapter 10

Materials

Principal Authors: Stanley E. Sagov, M.D., and Archie Brodsky

The materials required or recommended for home birth include everything necessary for the safety, comfort, and convenience of the mother and baby as well as the attendant. They range from familiar household items to emergency equipment and medications that are rarely, if ever, put to use. The provision of materials for the birth is another area in which responsibility is shared by the family and the attendant. Part of the family's preparation for the birth is to have specified materials on hand in readiness for the labor and delivery. Nonetheless, the attendant remains responsible for bringing to the home those items that are the tools of the practitioner's trade.

MATERIALS PROVIDED BY ATTENDANT

The attendant comes to the home equipped with a broad range of equipment, supplies, and pharmaceuticals designed to accommodate all anticipated needs of the mother and baby during a normal labor and delivery (allowing for the many variations of normality) as well as during any medical emergency that may be anticipated. The exact composition of the attendant's home birth kit will vary with the region and its governing professional norms, the attendant's training and qualifications, the nature of available support systems, the distance (in miles and minutes) from backup facilities, and the volume of births attended. For example, in countries where obstetric flying squads are trained to perform emergency procedures in specially equipped ambulances, it may not be necessary to bring such items as adult resuscitation equipment to the birth site. Even where flying squads do not exist, physicians and midwives may not need to carry a great deal of emergency equipment in areas where home birth is an accepted norm and hospital transfers are regarded as routine. Exam-

151

ples of the range of variation in different settings may be found in such sources as Myles[1] for Great Britain and Arms[2] for the Netherlands.

In the United States, where mobile backup is not available and the professional environment is not usually supportive of home birth, the home birth attendant is advised to approximate as closely as possible the capabilities of hospital obstetric and neonatal services. The following inventory of materials (grouped by function) represents an adaptation of the standard hospital delivery room in the Boston area to the portable form required for home delivery. It errs deliberately on the side of safety, particularly with regard to adult and infant resuscitation and neonatal support. Designed for use by a physician-midwife team, it contains drugs and other items whose availability to midwives working without physicians varies from state to state. Some items, such as umbilical artery catheters, are used in the home only in extremely rare instances, even by physicians, and should not be considered essential supplies. Although it is recognized that home birth attendants in the United States and elsewhere practice successfully with a small, "basic" birth kit, an inclusive supply list is provided here so that practitioners can exercise their own judgment concerning selection.

Vaginal Examination

- ovum forceps, 2 (to clean cervix and allow exposure of interior)
- Sims retractor, 1 (to allow exposure of interior)
- vaginal speculum (bivalve), 1
- sterile lubricant, 5 oz. (for speculum)
- sterile gloves, 6 pair

Fetal Heart Monitoring

- fetoscope, 1
- ultrasound monitor, 1
- ultrasound conducting solution, 8 oz.

Intrapartum and Postpartum Care

- adult stethoscope, 1
- sphygmomanometer (blood pressure cuff), 1
- oxygen tank (with adult face masks), 1
- oxygen refill, 1
- oral airway, adult, 1 (for oxygen)
- nitrazine® paper, 1 strip (to test ph of vaginal secretion)

- urinary catheter, French No. 14, 2 (to empty bladder)
- Amnihook®, 1 (for amniotomy)
- gauze pads, 4×4, 12 (for perineal support)
- silastic vacuum cup with pump, 1 (to extract baby when required)
- laryngoscope (with 2 bulbs, Nos. 0, 1, 3 Miller blades, 2 batteries), 1 (to examine airway)
- endotracheal catheters, Nos. 2.5, 3.0, 3.5, Cole or Portex type, 1 each (for resuscitation)
- epinephrine, 1:10,000, 10-ml cartridge (1 mg)
- meperidine (Demerol®), 1.0-ml ampules (50 mg), 4 (for emergency pain relief prior to transfer to hospital only)
- sodium bicarbonate, 50-ml cartridge (50 mEq)

Care of Umbilical Cord

- Kelly clamp, 1 (to clamp cord prior to cutting)
- curved scissors, 1 (to cut cord)
- cord clamp, 2 (to secure end of cord attached to baby)

Stimulation of Uterine Contractions Postpartum

- oxytocin (Pitocin®), 1.0-ml syringes (10 units), 4
- oxytocin (Pitocin®) ampules (10 units), 4
- methylergonovine (Methergine®), 1.0 ml (0.2 mg), 4
- ergonovine maleate (Ergotrate Maleate®) tablets, 0.2 mg, 100

Parenteral Medication (Injection)

- syringes, 1 ml with 25 gauge × ¾-inch needle, 3 ml with 22 gauge × 1½-inch needle, 4 each (for vitamin K and other medications)
- syringes, 10 ml (with control handle), 2 (for anesthesia)
- needles, 20-, 22-, and 25-gauge, 4 each
- alcohol pads, 4
- sterile water, 20 ml, 5 (to dilute medications)

Surgical Supplies for Episiotomy, Repair of Laceration, and Hemostasis

- sterile barrier field, 4 (to spread instruments)
- episiotomy scissors, 1
- gauze pads (to allow visualization of repair)

- towel clamp, 2 (for sterile field)
- toothed forceps, 1
- ovum forceps
- curved mosquito clamp, 4 (for hemostasis)
- needle holder, 2
- spinal needles, No. 22, 3½-inch, 4
- lidocaine (Xylocaine®), 1%, 50 ml (500 mg) (to anesthetize area)
- sterile specimen cup, 1 (to prepare lidocaine for injection)
- Ethicon® chromic sutures, 2-0 and 3-0, 2 each
- sterile gloves

Blood Drawing

- tourniquet (rubber tubing), 1
- Vacutainer® needles, No. 20, 1½-inch, 4
- Vacutainer® tube, 4
- lancets, 4 (to obtain blood from baby)
- Band-Aids, 4

Intravenous Therapy (Maternal)

- IV tubing kit, 2
- butterfly® needles, Nos. 19 and 21, 2 each
- adhesive tape, ½-inch, 1 roll
- angiocatheter, No. 18, 2
- Quick-Cath®, No. 20, 1¼-inch, 2
- normal saline, 20 ml
- lactated Ringer's solution, 1,000 ml
- normal serum albumin, 5%, 250 ml

Normal Newborn Care and Examination

- infant stethoscope, 1
- reflex hammer, 1
- otoscope-ophthalmoscope (with 2 bulbs, 2 batteries), 1
- tongue depressors, 10
- measuring tapes, paper, 10
- cord blood paper, 1 (for metabolic screen)
- worksheet for birth certificate, 1

- AquaMEPHYTON® solution (vitamin K$_1$), 4
- erythromycin eye ointment, 0.125 oz. (for venereal disease protection)
- silver nitrate ophthalmic solution, wax ampule, 1

Newborn Resuscitation

- oxygen tank
- oral airway, infant, 1 (for oxygen)
- Penlon-Cardiff ventilation bag (with masks), 1
- laryngoscope
- endotracheal tubes
- bulb syringe, 1 (to suction nose, mouth)
- DeLee suction catheter, 1 (to suction lungs)
- protocol for newborn resuscitation, 1
- atropine sulfate, 0.5-ml ampules (0.4 mg), 2
- calcium gluconate, 10-ml ampule (1 gm)
- sodium bicarbonate, 10-ml cartridge (20 mEq)
- dextrose, 50%, 50-ml syringe
- epinephrine

Umbilical Artery Catheterization

- scalpel with No. 15 blade
- iris forceps, 1 (to insert catheter)
- three-way stopcock
- umbilical artery catheters, Nos. 3.5 and 5F, 1 each
- infant feeding tube, No. 8F, 1
- heparin (Lipo-Hepin®), 10 ml (10,000 units) (to prevent blood clotting)
- sodium chloride

General

- veterinary-sized doctor's bag, 1
- plastic instrument tray, 1
- chlorhexidene gluconate (Hibiclens®), 4 oz.
- prescription pad, 1

With the exception of the hand-sized ultrasound monitor and the oxygen tank, all the materials listed can be carried in the veterinary-sized doctor's bag. The attendant(s) should institute a protocol for replacing materials consumed during each birth and regularly checking equipment for proper functioning and pharmaceuticals and sterilized items for expiration dates. The entire kit is autoclaved every three months. (See instructions for sterilization at the end of this chapter.)

Although some of the larger pieces of equipment entail a substantial capital investment for the independent practitioner, the cost of maintaining the kit is not high when calculated on a per-birth basis. For example, if the practitioners using the kit attend 60 births per year, and if all items are assumed to require replacement in a maximum of five years, the cost of materials is estimated to be approximately $15 per birth. If the volume of births is 120 per year, the cost per birth is approximately $10.[3]

The attendant should be aware that having a complete and up-to-date set of materials is just a first step. The attendant must exercise judgment concerning when to use the various items and maintain skill in using them. In some cases this may require proficiency in techniques that in the hospital are left to highly specialized personnel.

MATERIALS PROVIDED BY FAMILY

Families who choose to have a birth at home rather than in the prepared hospital environment assume the responsibility of getting their home ready for the birth. Most families gladly undertake to provide a safe and comfortable setting as part of their overall management of the birth. In the rare case when a family has failed to make the necessary preparations by the time the pregnancy reaches term, there may be grounds to reconsider the choice of a home birth.

Among the materials given to families planning a home birth is a list of supplies to be obtained and set aside for the birth. Since these materials must complement the attendant's home birth supply kit, the contents of the family's supply list will depend in part on what the attendant does or does not bring to the home. In the authors' practice families are instructed to have the following items on hand:

- chlorhexidene gluconate (Hibiclens®) antiseptic (for vaginal examinations, hand wash)
- nail brush (for cleaning hands—optional)
- witch hazel
- flashlight with new batteries
- mirror (optional)

- heating pad or hot water bottle
- wash cloths for compresses (to be kept hot in a crock pot or skillet)
- disposable underpads (1 dozen)
- thermometer
- fleet enema
- oil (vitamin E, coconut, olive, sesame) for perineum, small unopened bottle
- bowl (large, for placenta)
- sanitary belt
- sanitary napkins, regular and hospital size
- tape measure
- alcohol (for cord care)
- packaged sterile supplies:
  cotton balls (for cord care)
  gauze pads, 4 × 4 (2 dozen)
  gloves, disposable, sizes 7½, 8 (6 pair each size)
- sterile equipment, to be boiled for 30 minutes:
  scissors
  cord clamps or sterile white shoelaces (2)
  bulb syringe with soft rubber tip, 3-oz. size (sold as ear syringe)
  tongs (to lift sterile items from water—optional)

The instructions for families state that after the sterile equipment has been boiled (which may be done ahead of time), the scissors and cord clamps are to be kept in a covered dish. The bulb syringe may be wrapped in a soft sterile cloth.

The surface on which the birth is to take place should be protected. A bed, for example, should be made with two sets of clean sheets separated by a layer of rubber or plastic. After the birth the top layer of sheets is taken off along with the rubber or plastic. Underpads should be used beneath the bottom layer of sheets since there will be some postpartum bleeding. Bloodstained sheets can easily be cleaned by soaking in cold water.

It will be noted that several items (e.g., Hibiclens, gauze pads, gloves, cord clamps, bulb syringe) are included in both the attendant's and the family's supply lists. In these instances the attendant's supplies serve a backup function, so that essential procedures may be performed even if the family's supplies are depleted. Having the family provide these easily obtained consumer goods reduces the attendant's operating expenses and increases the family's sense of involvement. For poor families, however, the attendant may wish to furnish these items. Families also can reduce or defray the cost of materials by making use of existing household supplies wherever possible; finding other household uses for materials left over from the birth; and obtaining unused materials from other families in the childbirth classes.

WHERE TO OBTAIN MATERIALS

Equipment and supplies for the attendant are available from mail order houses specializing in materials for home birth. Some of the same centers stock birth supplies for families as well as baby carriers, herbs, and oils (see Appendix B).

METHODS OF STERILIZATION

All nondisposable instruments must be sterilized between deliveries. There are several acceptable methods of sterilization either at or before a birth.

At the Birth

Instruments may be sterilized by one of the following methods:

1. Prewashed instruments are placed in a pot that is filled with cold water above the level of the instruments. The water is brought to a boil. After the water has continued to boil for 30 minutes, the lid is opened slightly so that the water can be poured out while the instruments are held in the pot. The pot is again covered tightly and the instruments allowed to cool. The insides of the pot and lid can be considered sterile for 12 hours, after which the instruments should be resterilized if the birth has not yet occurred. (Although widely used, this is probably not as effective an antiseptic method as those listed below.)
2. Prewashed and prewrapped instruments are baked at 250 degrees for 1 hour and used when cool.
3. Instruments are soaked for 30 minutes in formaldehyde germicide or Glutarex® (active ingredient: glutaraldchyde) disinfecting and sterilizing solution.

Before the Birth

Instruments may be sterilized in advance by any of the three methods listed above. After cooling, instruments are placed in sealable plastic bags with sterile tongs and stored in the birth kit until needed. Instruments may also be autoclaved or sterilized in a pressure cooker under 15 pounds pressure for 30 minutes.

Sterilized instruments should be double wrapped in either sterilization paper or clean linen squares. They are then taped and dated. Instruments must be resterilized if the wrapping becomes wet or torn.

NOTES

1. Margaret F. Myles, *Textbook for Midwives*, 8th ed. (Edinburgh: Churchill Livingstone, 1975), pp. 621–624.

2. Suzanne Arms, *Immaculate Deception; A New Look at Women and Childbirth in America* (Boston: Houghton Mifflin, 1975).

3. Mary Lee Ingbar et al., "Choosing Services for Maternity Care and Childbirth: A Case Study" (Worcester, Mass.: University of Massachusetts Medical School, Department of Family and Community Medicine, 1980), pp. III, 69.

Chapter 11

Labor and Delivery

Principal Authors: Peggy Spindel, R.N., and Stanley E. Sagov, M.D.

This chapter will focus on the management of normal labor in the home, with emphasis on the timely detection of abnormalities to allow for a smooth transfer to the hospital or—in rare cases in which the speed of events does not allow for a transfer—emergency management at home. Our discussion assumes a basic knowledge of the physiology and mechanisms of labor and the availability of textbooks that deal more exhaustively with the complications mentioned. This outline of the conduct of labor is neither encyclopedic nor absolutely prescriptive on all points. Rather, it represents a distillation of the authors' experience in managing labors both at home and in the hospital. Since the proper conduct of labor is not site dependent, the approach described is applicable in the hospital or out-of-hospital birth center as well as the home.

Nonetheless, the definition of the normal course of labor is a major source of disagreement between practitioners who favor hospital delivery and those who favor home delivery. In general, obstetric attendants in teaching institutions whose view of labor comes from receiving referrals of complicated cases may be more likely to apply textbook guidelines strictly and to have a lower threshold for active management. Those who regularly attend home births, on the other hand, being highly sensitized to their clients' desire for individualistic, holistic care, may be able to learn from experience how enormous variations in patterns of labor can result in the desired outcome of a healthy mother and baby. Thus, although it is useful for purposes of both teaching and practice to subdivide labor into stages and to set approximate time limits for their completion, in the absence of maternal or fetal distress home birth attendants are generally reluctant to intervene to achieve an arbitrary numerical rate of progress when labor is in fact progressing (albeit slowly).

The management of labor at home requires considerable clinical skill because of the reduced availability of the technical resources found in the hospital. There is less margin for error. To obtain the necessary information and make the necessary judgments, one must blend the obstetrician's science with the midwife's art—or, looked at in another way, practice a twentieth-century, probabilistic science of clinical decision making that includes an awareness of uncertainty and intangible factors heretofore relegated to "the art of medicine."[1] The experienced attendant learns to respect the way the process of labor has evolved to ensure survival of the human species and yet be attuned to those clinical observations that dictate prompt action for diagnosis or treatment. The attendant must distinguish between variations of labor that are merely inconvenient for the attendant or institution and variations that portend a bad outcome for the mother or baby.

The home birth attendant's characteristic stance is unobtrusive. Most women who have been screened and prepared as outlined in previous chapters (and many who have not) can deliver successfully with the natural support of family and friends. A laboring woman should, therefore, be able to feel safe from unnecessary intervention, anxiety, or control on the part of the attendant. Yet the attendant must be a watchful observer, objectively reviewing what has taken place, what is presently happening, and what problems (if any) can be anticipated. Furthermore, in difficult labors the attendant must be prepared to give the woman and family intense devotion and added creative energy.

Finally, the attendant must know the limits of his or her own competence and must be prepared to make judgments concerning when to seek help and when to move to the hospital for completion of the labor and delivery. Barriers to timely transfer include emotional identification with the home site, reluctance to disappoint or come into conflict with the family, and fear of adverse criticism resulting from exposing one's errors to hospital personnel. At the other extreme, fear of bad outcomes and of censure from colleagues can lead to an overcautious approach, resulting in unnecessary transfers. Still, the inexperienced attendant whose clinical intuition is not yet highly developed would do better to err in the direction of safety. When transfer is indicated, the attendant must exert moral leadership by helping the family adopt a more reasonable course of action than their initial emotional reactions might dictate. It is always possible to return to the home if consultations and diagnostic evaluations in the hospital yield reassuring indications about the progress of labor and the well-being of the mother and baby.

THE APPROACH OF LABOR

Signs and Symptoms

The signs and symptoms of approaching labor include "lightening," "ripening" of the cervix, increased Braxton-Hicks contractions, rupture of the membranes, bloody show, spurts of energy, and diarrhea or other gastrointestinal upsets. Other signs include sensations such as achiness or congestion in the pelvic area, feeling "premenstrual," increased swelling or heaviness in the vulva, shooting pains or cramps in the upper legs, and a feeling of increased pressure on the cervix. All these changes are related to the descent of the presenting part and the contractions of the uterus in preparation for labor.

These early changes help prepare both the woman and the attendant for the onset of labor. Most women welcome the end of pregnancy and use the last few days to be sure everything and everyone is prepared. The woman should be reminded to take it easy and to eat well, being especially careful to take in at least 300 calories a day above her nonpregnant daily requirement. The baby will soon be born, and the mother needs to conserve her energy. Some women need reassurance that the signs listed above are all normal and in fact are positive indicators of the body's proper functioning.

Emotional Issues

Approaching labor can bring out or intensify fears about the birth process or the new baby. The attendant should be alert and available for this last opportunity to work through these anxieties before labor begins. Some useful steps include the following:

- practicing relaxation techniques learned in prenatal classes
- meditation
- visualization exercises[2]
- dinner out or a glass of wine, a hot bath, a backrub, or other loving contact with partner
- contact with supportive prospective grandparents or supportive peers with newborns
- avoidance of contact with anxiety-provoking stimuli such as unsupportive prospective grandparents or friends with birth "horror stories"
- clearing up fears related to previous births, abortions, or miscarriages. Often the physical sensations of late pregnancy will reactivate these worries.

Clinical Review

In a planned home birth, information about general health, past and present pregnancies, patterns of past labors, and risk factors that may impact upon the management of labor will already have been obtained. These data should be reviewed by the attendant when the woman reports signs of approaching labor. The attendant should consult the record to be sure that the pregnancy is still low risk, that the baby is of appropriate size, and that the pregnancy is neither preterm nor prolonged. No potentially serious clinical issues or contradictions in the data should be left unresolved.

Conditions Requiring Further Evaluation

High Presenting Part. Check (especially in primigravida) for overlap of the head in front of the pubic bone, which may indicate cephalopelvic disproportion (CPD), although this sign should not be regarded as decisive.[3]

Borderline Prematurity. Occasionally a home birth at 36½ weeks with a good-sized baby and a mother with a short menstrual cycle will be considered by some midwives on the basis of anecdotal experience.

Postmaturity. Postmaturity should be dealt with by criteria developed with consultants and consistent with local standards (see discussion in Chapter 5). Risk assessment can be refined by review of prenatal monitoring.

Frank Bleeding and/or Sudden Severe Abdominal Pain. Do not perform vaginal examination. Rule out placenta previa with ultrasound and obstetric consultation when appropriate. Rule out abruptio placentae, appendicitis, or other causes of abdominal pain.

Premature Rupture of the Membranes. If the membranes are thought to be ruptured, the woman should be examined as soon as possible. (If it is in the middle of the night, and if the baby's head is low, the fluid clear, and the baby normally active, the father can be asked to listen to the baby's heart with the ear alone or with the aid of an empty toilet paper roll against the abdomen. If all seems well, the woman can be seen by the attendant in the morning.)

If there is any sign of complication (e.g., if the baby's head is not low, the fluid not clear, or the baby not normally active), the woman should go to bed and should be visited by the attendant immediately. A digital examination should not be performed unless there is a question of a prolapsed cord. If it is not clear whether rupture has taken place at all, a sterile vaginal speculum examination can be done, checking for fluid coming from the os with or without fundal pressure, nitrazine positive fluid, or "ferning" of collected fluid under a microscope.

If premature rupture of the membranes is either confirmed or probable, the following surveillance measures should be taken:

1. Fetal heart tones are monitored every two to four hours by the attendant or parents. The normal range is 120 to 160 beats per minute. A rising baseline fetal heart rate may be indicative of infection.
2. Maternal temperature and pulse are taken every two to four hours. Readings up to 99°F and 90 beats per minute are considered normal.
3. White blood cell counts and differentials are obtained daily. Review results with consultant if questionable.
4. The mother is instructed not to engage in sexual intercourse, not to douche or put anything, such as a tampon, in her vagina, and to maintain good genital hygiene. She should avoid the continuous use of sanitary napkins. She should eat well, drink plenty of fluids, and get as much rest as possible. Tub baths should be avoided, but showers are permissible. The parents should be alerted to the suddenness with which serious infection can occur, and the risks in proceeding with the home birth should be discussed again under these changed circumstances. Phone contact with the attendant should be frequent and any contractions noted.
5. If the baseline fetal heart rate increases by as much as 5 to 10 beats per minute, have the mother push fluids (eight ounces per hour) and rest. The tachycardia may be due simply to maternal dehydration and may be correctable. If the fetal heart rate does not return to baseline but all other indicators remain normal, give the mother castor oil and monitor her very carefully. (See instructions for castor oil induction later in this chapter.) A "stat" white blood cell count is useful here. If the woman does not then go into labor, a consultation is obtained and a transfer to the hospital is considered. If there is maternal tachycardia (greater than 90 beats per minute), fever (above 99°F), uterine tenderness, or purulent discharge, then a transfer should be made.[4] If the white blood cell count rises above normal limits, with increased band forms, a consultation is needed. The attendant should be alert for signs of septic shock, which may occur very suddenly.

Although it is common practice in hospitals to induce labor in cases of premature rupture of the membranes with a full-term baby, the value of induction in such cases is not documented. It is the authors' belief that the risk of infection for a well-nourished woman at term who remains in her own home does not mandate the transfer to hospital that is required for induction. The danger of infection *is*, however, increased by prolonged labor, excessive vaginal examinations, exhaustion, and dehydration, and these are to be scrupulously avoided.

THE ONSET OF LABOR

In a home birth the "diagnosis" or determination of the onset of labor is necessary, not to admit the woman to the labor and delivery floor of a hospital but to know when she is ready for constant attendance and frequent monitoring. Yet the onset of labor may be so gradual as to defy definition and may in retrospect have to be somewhat arbitrarily assigned to a given time.

Initial Phone Contact

Clients should be asked to call when they think that labor is beginning or when contractions are approximately 5 minutes apart for a primipara or 10 minutes apart for a multipara. The woman should come to the phone, and the attendant should listen to her through a contraction. The attendant can begin to assess whether and how far advanced the woman is in labor on the basis of how she responds to the contraction (e.g., whether she continues to talk in a normal manner).

The woman should be seen if any of the following conditions are found:

- mild contractions 5 minutes apart, lasting 30 seconds or longer, and bloody show
- strong contractions 5 minutes apart even without bloody show
- possible rupture of membranes and a high head as noted on the last prenatal examination (check color of fluid)
- inability of woman to come to the phone
- in the case of multipara with history of short labors—as soon as she calls

If the prospective parents cannot give a clear history, they should be asked to keep an accurate record for an hour and call back. If there is an obvious emergency such as a cord prolapse or heavy bleeding, the attendant should arrange to meet the couple at the hospital rather than waste time going to the home. If no serious problem is detected at the hospital, the woman need not be admitted.

Initial Assessment of Labor

Before leaving for the home, the attendant should check the birth kit for completeness, briefly review the woman's record, and make sure of the directions to the home. On arrival, the attendant can place the birth kit in a convenient but not too obtrusive location and observe the labor for a while to get a sense of the pace of the contractions, the mood of the people present, and the functioning of the home. Whether or not the woman is in labor, this observation can yield information useful for interpreting later developments or initiating early corrective action. If the woman appears to be in active labor, the baby's heart rate should be listened to immediately, with further monitoring carried out according to the stage of labor.

Evaluation of Environment

Is it beneficial or counterproductive to the woman's peace of mind? Is any logistical support missing? Are any unhealthful activities (e.g., smoking) going on? Does the family have a functioning automobile (borrowed if necessary) available?

Evaluation of Contractions

Intensity, duration, and frequency of contractions along with a normal gradient pattern should be noted.

Fetal Heart and Fetal Presentation and Position

If there are any minor risk factors such as marginal prematurity or postmaturity, a brief auditory "nonstress test" can be done to assess the fetoplacental unit. Fetal heart tones are auscultated for 5 to 10 minutes. When an acceleration (in response to fetal movements) of 15 beats per minute occurs and lasts for more than 10 seconds, the test is considered reactive.[5] Although a single such acceleration is sufficient to reach this finding, the attendant may wish to listen for up to 15 minutes if fetal activity is good. Any other indications of fetal distress, particularly in relation to contractions, should also be noted. (See later section of this chapter on fetal distress.)

Assessment of the Mother

Extent of assessment, which may range from vital signs to full physical examination, will depend on the mother's apparent condition, stage of labor, and how well known she is to the attendant. The woman's response to her contractions, her attitude toward the impending birth, and other aspects of her emotional state should be assessed, along with how well her male partner is coping.

Pelvic Assessment

Pelvic assessment is to be done if the woman appears to be in labor and her membranes appear to be intact. The following should be checked:

- effacement
- dilatation
- station
- orientation of the cervix (e.g., anterior or posterior)
- status of membranes
- confirmation of position of baby
- presence of moulding and/or caput
- degree of relaxation of the pelvic floor and thighs and ease of examination (an indicator of how relaxed the woman will be for the delivery and how much perineal massage may be necessary)

Any changes (e.g., in dilatation, station) during a contraction should be noted. The attendant should take care to be gentle.

Sharing of Findings

Findings should be shared with the woman and her family or other support persons.

If the woman is not yet in active labor, is reasonably comfortable, and the environment is restful, the attendant may decide to leave the home. The attendant should remind the woman how to keep in good condition during this period (e.g., rest, fluids, light food, frequent urination, not too much heavy breathing or other forced labor techniques) and stress positive aspects of the ripening of the cervix and advancing signs and symptoms of prelabor. The parents-to-be should be instructed to call again at a time (estimated by the length and frequency of contractions) when clinical labor is deemed likely to have begun.

If the situation is at all unclear, either because the family is anxious or the clinical picture is confused, the attendant should stay until it is clarified. The couple may need a great deal of reassurance, especially if the woman is in pain and the cervix is only dilated 2 cm. Moreover, since true labor is always a retrospective diagnosis after a progressive dilatation of the cervix has occurred, there is sometimes legitimate uncertainty in the face of ambiguous indications that labor has begun. This ambiguity is especially marked when false labor is occurring.

False labor is more common in multiparous women. The contractions in false labor sometimes are distinguishable from those in true labor. They are felt much more in the front than in the back. They tend to be incoordinate in that they do not have a mild onset, peak, and then fall off in intensity. They last for longer than a minute, and they do not occur at periodic intervals. They are much more frequent at night or when lying down and are generally relieved by the ingestion of small amounts of alcohol or a relaxing hot bath. The presence of show, which tends not to occur with false labor, is a probable sign of the imminent onset of true labor, although a recent vaginal examination within a few days may make this sign unreliable, since the mucus plug may have been disturbed by the examining fingers.

When leaving the home of a woman who is experiencing contractions but is found not yet to be in labor, the attendant should encourage the family to be responsible for assessing themselves. The parents can monitor the fetal heart tones every one to two hours if the attendant leaves them a fetoscope. The woman should continue to feel that she is competent to interpret her own body sensations. Dependence on the birth attendant at this stage will make it harder for the woman to cope later. The father should be encouraged to have close physical contact with the mother, either through simple touching or through massage, so that he can strengthen his nonverbal knowledge of the mother and his ability to interpret her needs. Sometimes another family member such as a sister may be good at this kind of contact, while the father may be more comfortable in another role. If the woman does not want to be touched by anyone, even in early labor, the attendants and family members or friends will have to learn to "read" her in other ways. A family that is in good communication with the laboring woman can be relied on to make a timely call to the attendant when the woman needs to be seen again.

OVERVIEW OF LABOR

Labor is traditionally divided into three stages, with a fourth recently proposed. The first stage is that of cervical dilatation, lasting from the onset of contractions to full dilatation. This stage is further divided into a latent phase and an active phase, the demarcation point occurring at a dilatation of 3 to 4 cm. The second stage begins at full dilatation and ends with the birth of the baby. The third stage is that of separation and expulsion of the placenta and membranes. In order to promote heightened vigilance in the immediate postpartum period, the first hour after the delivery of the placenta is now commonly designated as the fourth stage of labor.

A woman in labor at home should be continuously supported and monitored by a qualified attendant from the beginning of active labor. In addition, it is recommended that a second attendant come to the home before the transition to the second stage. Although some home birth attendants do work alone, there have been several occasions in the authors' experience when the presence of a second attendant has been crucial to a successful outcome. The practice of working in pairs allows for the inevitable fluctuations of energy in a long labor, increases the likelihood of timely correction of errors, and provides an opportunity for discussion among knowledgeable people in the case of diagnostic uncertainty in evaluating progress or in recognizing potential abnormalities. Two people are far better able than one to respond adequately to an emerging crisis, especially when the mother and baby require simultaneous attention.

If the person monitoring the labor from the beginning is a qualified assistant, the primary attendant should plan to arrive *no later than* 6 cm of dilatation for a primigravida and 4 cm for a multigravida. The midwife or physician who will be there for the delivery should be with the woman long enough to know the flow of her labor, her laboring style, and her physical and psychological needs. Family members, friends, or others invited just for the birth should be called no later than 8 to 10 cm of dilatation for a primigravida and 4 to 6 cm for a multigravida (depending on effacement and station), subject to the character of the labor.

PROBLEMS IN LATENT PHASE

Even before active labor begins, serious problems requiring immediate attention may occur. The attendant should be alert for the following complications as manifested in early labor:

1. *frank bleeding*. A vaginal examination should not be done. Since a heavy show at the start of dilatation may not be indicative of further problems, some attendants believe it unnecessary to transfer the woman to the hospital if the bleeding stops quickly and does not resume. If the fetal heart tones are good and bleeding is moderate, these attendants regard it as sufficient to listen to the baby very frequently and to monitor the mother's pulse and blood pressure. Their experience notwithstanding, it is generally regarded as more acceptable to transfer the woman in all cases of frank bleeding. If placenta previa and other serious complications are able to be ruled out, returning to the home may be considered.

2. *frank bleeding with poor or absent fetal heart tones*. An IV is started prior to transfer by ambulance to closest hospital. The mother is

placed in a lateral position and given oxygen until the ambulance arrives.

3. *cord prolapse*. An ambulance should be called immediately. The cord is replaced in the vagina if it appears at the vulva. With a sterile glove on, push the fetal head gently upward to relieve the pressure on the cord until the surgeon lifts the baby out at the cesarean section, which is the usual method of delivery of a live baby after prolapse. If the cord is pinched between the symphysis and the head, the cord is moved gently to the side. Circulation can return to a flaccid cord if the pressures are relieved. The mother is placed in the knee-chest position while keeping a hand on the baby's head. (Alternately, the mother can be placed laterally in the Trendelenburg position by elevating the foot of the bed with bricks or books and/or placing pillows underneath her body.) The mother is given oxygen. Since this is an emergency transfer, the closest hospital should be called and should prepare for immediate surgery.

4. *breech position*. If the woman is in early labor, transfer to the hospital known for handling breeches most flexibly is advised.

5. *meconium fluid.*[6] If the fluid is lightly stained, if the fetal heart tones are good, and if no other risk factors (such as postmaturity) are present, an auditory "nonstress test" is done and the woman is followed closely at home. If the fluid is lightly stained but other risk factors are present, a transfer to hospital is in order. The baby's pediatrician (if other than the attendant) is alerted so that the parents will have an advocate for the baby in the hospital. If there is heavy meconium and poor fetal heart tones, transfer by ambulance, giving the mother oxygen, is done. However, if the fetal heart tones are good, despite heavy meconium, a nonemergent transfer to the hospital of choice can be considered (if time allows). Since heavy meconium may be indicative of a breech presentation, abdominal and vaginal findings should be included in the assessment.

ACTIVE LABOR IN THE FIRST STAGE

The birth attendant or a responsible assistant should be in the home throughout active labor (defined as at least 3 to 4 cm dilatation with contractions). The attendant should prepare the necessary equipment for labor monitoring but avoid making the home look like a hospital. The birth kit should be organized so that if the mother delivers suddenly, essential supplies will be accessible. The mother's supplies should be organized to suit the attendant's habits. The emergency phone list should be rechecked for currency and legibility. Instruments that are not presterilized should be boiled or otherwise sterilized in early active labor. The attendant should stay within earshot of the laboring woman, but not undertake direct labor support unless asked or unless necessary for other reasons.

Guidelines for Monitoring

Fetal and Maternal Vital Signs

The fetal heart tones should be monitored every 15 to 30 minutes during early active labor and every 5 to 15 minutes in late active labor (i.e., the transition to the second stage). (Note that this recommendation deviates slightly from those made by Haverkamp and associates[7] and Check.[8]) Particular attention is paid to transitional periods or times when the mother is anxious or stressed. To get an idea of the variability of the fetal heart rate, one can count for 15 seconds three or four times, multiplying each result by four (or count for 10 seconds several times, multiplying by six). The heart rate can vary within the range of 120 to 160 beats per minute. Within this broad range there will be a baseline around which the heart rate should show a short-term variation of 5 to 10 beats per minute. (True beat-to-beat variation is probably not reliably audible.) The baseline will also show a long-term variation within the overall range of 120 to 160 beats per minute. These normal variations are an indication of fetal well-being.[9] From time to time the baby should be listened to throughout a contraction and directly afterward to evaluate the baby's response to and recovery from the stress of the contraction. (See later section of this chapter on fetal distress.)

A baseline blood pressure reading of the mother, as well as pulse and temperature, should be taken in early labor. If indicated, they should be repeated every two to four hours.

Vaginal Examinations

Deciding when to do a vaginal examination is an art in itself. Instead of strict protocols there are two general indications: (1) the attendant's need to know to monitor progress and diagnose problems and /or (2) the mother's need to know for reassurance and interest. A vaginal examination may need to be performed under the following conditions:

- at the beginning of active contractions—to establish the onset and stage of labor and to find out if the baby might come very quickly (e.g., 100 percent effacement, 4-cm dilatation, head at +1 station, bulging membranes in multipara)

- at the end of the first stage—to confirm other signs of full dilatation, including the mother's urge to push
- to ascertain the reason for an apparent arrest of progress at any stage
- to rule out cord prolapse immediately after rupture of the membranes
- to predict the time of birth so as to time the arrival of other attendants

In a normal labor one or two vaginal examinations may suffice. Because of the risk of infection, the use of sterile gloves and an antiseptic solution such as Betadine® or Hibiclens® or a sterile lubricant is mandatory. Hibiclens is preferable because its color allows it to be distinguished from meconium more readily than Betadine. Once the membranes have ruptured, it is even more important to limit the number of examinations in the interest of preventing infection.

As long as a vaginal examination is indicated, despite the discomfort and disruption often experienced by laboring women, it is important to do a complete examination so that the information can be accurate and useful. After each examination the examiner should be able to report findings in all of the categories listed above under Initial Assessment of Labor. Documentation of these findings in the record allows for objective assessments of progress that can be used either to reassure anxious participants in the birth process or (if necessary) to explain the decision to transfer.

During a vaginal examination the attendant should help the laboring woman relax as much as possible by maintaining verbal and eye contact when appropriate. If a contraction occurs during the examination, it is valuable to note what happens to the station of the presenting part and whether or not the membranes are bulging. It is also important to recognize that the increased stress of the contraction requires one to be more gentle and to stay in place, rather than continue to probe, until the contraction has passed.

Observations Requiring Further Evaluation

The following observations may simply indicate that the woman needs more intense labor support or that the second stage is approaching. However, they can also be early indications of complications. The last two groups of signs in particular have significant diagnostic implications.

1. rapid breathing, especially between contractions
2. clenched fists or other muscle tension or writhing or thrashing
3. expressions of fear, inability to maintain eye contact, unusual worry about the baby, lack of suggestibility, marked increase in pain unrelated to contractions (e.g., pain in legs, headache, chest pain), loss

of support from male partner, desire to go to the hospital, refusal to cooperate with attendants or family, and inability to get enough rest to get ready for the next contraction
4. poor skin turgor, sunken eyeballs, dry lips, ketones in urine, pulse over 90, temperature over 99°F. Given any of these findings, check fetal heart tones for rising baseline.
5. increased edema, especially in face or hands, blood pressure over 140/90 (or 15 mm Hg over prenatal levels), change in level of consciousness, jitteriness, hyperreflexia, headache, epigastric pain, visual disturbances, sense of constriction of the thorax,[10] protein in the urine greater than a trace, oliguria. Given any of these findings, check for ankle clonus. Hold the woman's flexed leg with one hand under the knee. With the other hand, sharply dorsiflex her foot and hold it in a flexed position. Her foot will jerk against the attendant's hand one or more times if clonus is present. Clonus may indicate that there is preeclampsia with central nervous system involvement.[11]

The key to assessing the seriousness of these observations is serial examinations and the presence of a fully elaborated syndrome as opposed to isolated symptoms. Particularly in the case of the signs in group 4 (indicating possible infection) or group 5 (indicating possible preeclampsia), any one of the findings listed should alert the attendant to look carefully for others in the same category. If an entire syndrome is found, transfer to the hospital is mandatory.

Home Environment

Finally, the home environment should be monitored throughout the labor. A good environment includes the following:

• peacefulness
• flexibility
• good organization
• appropriate focus on the labor
• phone answered or calls stopped
• soothing music or quiet
• no demands made on the mother
• support of children when necessary[12]

If the atmosphere is tense, the attendant, who may be the only one with any idea about how to smooth things out, should not hesitate to make suggestions.

Physical and Personal Needs of the Laboring Woman

Many people choose home birth so that they can be free to walk around in a familiar environment and to have access to food and drink as well as other personal conveniences. The attendant should treat the home environment as a valuable resource and help the woman go through labor as comfortably as possible.

Food in Labor

Obstetricians as a rule regard the ingestion of solid food in labor as unsafe and ineffective. Any food or fluid in the stomach increases the danger of aspiration should general (or even high spinal) anesthesia be required. Since it cannot be predicted with certainty in any given case that anesthesia will not be used, it is common practice to deny all laboring women any oral intake prophylactically. Should labor last long enough so that additional calories and fluid are needed for bodily functioning, these must be supplied intravenously. Those who follow this policy generally do so in the belief that digestion and absorption usually stop in labor anyway and the ingestion of food is therefore likely to be followed by vomiting.

Most midwives, physicians, and childbirth educators experienced with home birth believe otherwise. Women in their own homes have been found to tolerate moderate food intake, especially in latent or early active labor. Home birth attendants therefore claim that it is fear, more than labor, that stops digestion, and that vomiting is not necessarily related to food in the stomach. This divergence from standard obstetric practice should be discussed prenatally so that the family can make an informed choice regarding the risk of aspiration.

In a population of normal women experiencing natural childbirth in their own homes, the incidence of general anesthesia (following transfer to hospital) is very low. However, since anesthesia occasionally is required, obstetric backup personnel for home births should be familiar with techniques for preventing aspiration under general anesthesia (such as endotracheal intubation with a cuffed tube, the use of atropine and an antacid prior to induction, or the use of the Sellick maneuver to occlude the esophagus).[13]

Certain categories of foods are better tolerated than others by the woman in labor. Easily digested carbohydrates such as bread, fruit, rice, or pasta and light proteins such as cheese or yogurt can be taken as long as the woman wants them. As labor progresses, the emphasis should change to high-calorie liquids. Water, "athletic" drinks such as Gatorade®, iced tea, and noncitrus fruit juices are well tolerated. Straight honey or sugar will provide calories for the woman who wants to drink plain water. Eight ounces of fluid and 200 calories an hour are optimal. A tablespoon of honey contains 64 calories;[14] one cup of grape juice yields 167 calories.[15] Others at the birth, especially the father, should remember to eat and drink as well, since their support and energy will be required.

It is the experience of some attendants that citrus and apple juices and dairy products can cause vomiting in heavy labor. Some women freeze juices such as cranberry or grape in ice trays to use in the event of nausea. The crushed ice from juice, ice chips, or small sips of cool water are kept down if taken in small amounts between each contraction. Dry toast is also used in this manner.

A woman who pushes fluids in labor should also urinate frequently (at one to two-hour intervals) to avoid damage to an overfilled bladder and (although only in rare cases[16]) obstruction of labor. The woman may need to be reminded to do so, since the sensations of labor may mask the urge to urinate. Inadequate nutrition during labor is manifested by ketones in the urine (greater than trace), lack of energy, feelings of discouragement, signs of dehydration (e.g., dry lips, tachycardia, reduced urine output), and even uterine inertia. If a woman knows that it is *essential* for her to take in more fluid and calories, she usually can find something she can digest. Early attention to food and drink is the key to preventing prolonged labor due to dehydration or ketosis.

Position and Movement

There is evidence that a vertical position and ambulation improve the quality and effectiveness of labor and reduce the pain of uterine contraction, thereby shortening the first stage of labor.[17-22] The attendant can therefore encourage the woman to walk around during labor and to experiment with different positions, both as a way of feeling in control and as a device for coping with pain. However, a woman who is up and about should also have periods of rest.

Labor Support

Labor support is really only a matter of human beings meeting human needs and as such cannot easily be prescribed. However, the attendant should be ready with suggestions, especially to families who are inexperienced with birth.

Frequently a prospective father, after attending classes and reading books, complains to the attendant at the end of the pregnancy that he still does not have a sense of what he is supposed to do. One suggestion might be that he think about how he usually shows his mate that he loves her and then do just that. Likewise, labor support by anyone should be personal and consistent with that particular relationship.

Labor Support as Performed by the Woman in Labor

Much labor support consists simply of things that the woman in labor does for herself. Such activities may include the following:

- position changes—support with pillows or people
- movement—pelvic rock, free-form dancing and swaying
- self-massage—abdominal effleurage
- application of heat and cold—heat on lower abdomen, small of back, sacrum, between thighs, perineum; cold on face, neck, chest, sacrum; use of fan if hot
- grooming—hair brushing, toothbrushing
- attention to pleasing odors—flowers, perfumes, food, other essences such as pine or bay
- going outside—walking, sitting on porch, swinging in hammock, shopping, going to a movie
- listening to music or watching television
- water activities—bathtub, shower, shampoo
- meditation or visualization techniques
- relaxation exercises
- labor breathing—prepared (Lamaze, Bradley, American Society for Psychoprophylaxis in Obstetrics (ASPO)—see Appendix A) or made up on the spot
- singing, humming, playing an instrument
- mental techniques such as counting, clock watching
- knitting or sewing

Labor Support as Performed by Others

Labor support on the part of the male partner, family, friends, and the attendant supplements the support the woman gives herself. Labor support is based on physical contact and emotional closeness, with the male partner frequently playing the central role. Some typical forms of contact and closeness are as follows:

- massage of abdomen, face, brow, back of head, shoulders, neck, back, sacrum (particularly steady pressure during a contraction[23]), sacroiliac joints, hips and iliac crests, inner thighs, upper thighs, feet, or hands. A laboring woman often wants to be massaged by several people at once. Cornstarch is a good massage powder.
- breathing with the woman (or at least helping her keep her breathing relaxed)
- holding and supporting. The woman may want to walk around between contractions and then go limp during contraction. Some women also like to be held and cuddled during labor.
- verbal encouragement. Many women look particularly beautiful and glowing in active labor but think that they must look a mess. Positive feedback about the woman's appearance is helpful. Praise of all kinds is useful unless it embarrasses the woman. A woman in labor may enjoy hearing relaxing scenes or images described. It is essential to keep the woman focused on the present—the current contractions or rest period. Sometimes a woman may need to become more passive, dependent, or childlike in order to let go of the drive to know, to plan, and to control. The best person for her to lean on at such moments is her husband or male partner. The second best is probably her mother.
- eye contact—important for many women in order to feel connected emotionally with a support person. For other women, eye contact prevents them from letting go sufficiently to follow their instincts.
- application of heat and cold
- verbal and tactile relaxation techniques

Other supportive roles include cooking for all present, washing dishes, cleaning, answering the phone and doorbell, taking care of children and relatives, and shopping or running errands.

Creating an Atmosphere

Another form of labor support is to identify and help create different types of atmospheres, or environments, that support the mother's mood or answer her needs at different stages of the birth. Here are some examples:

- *festive*—lots of friends present, socializing, eating, enjoying music, with the mother joining in conversation between contractions. This is good for passing time and good for births with siblings. However, people become tired and demoralized if the birth does not come quickly. Sometimes people start to ignore the mother's needs, and she either becomes anxious or has to withdraw from others in order to focus on her labor.

- *resting*—darkened room, shades drawn, candles at night, very quiet, gentle massage of mother, slow relaxed breathing, mother in resting position with lots of pillows. Mood may become stagnated, or the woman may experience increased pain while lying down.
- *water*—hot bathtub (or shower), womblike dark quiet bathroom, washcloth over mother's eyes or her ears under water to reduce stimuli, one person for company who might trickle water over her abdomen during contractions. This is excellent for all types of labor but contraindicated with ruptured membranes (pending further investigation). The fetal heart can be heard through the water.
- *movement*—mother walking or dancing, lots of people for physical support, source of music, furniture out of the way to provide ample room for movement
- *intimate*—the mother-to-be and father-to-be alone together in an intense interpersonal experience. Some labors are always in this one-to-one mode, but the "significant other" changes shifts as people get tired.

Sometimes, even though the tone of the environment is consistent, it is simply time for a change. Often all that is needed is to remind the mother to urinate because she will naturally find something new when she gets out of the bathroom.

Change may be needed in the following instances:

- mother starts complaining
- general mood is restless
- sun rises or sets
- people come or go
- after meals
- when progress is poor
- at natural transition points in the labor
- when the mother has a premature urge to push

The last indication requires intervention by the attendant. Premature voluntary expulsive efforts by the laboring woman increase the risks of cervical lacerations, edema of the cervix, and stretching of uterine supports, which may actually impede the progress of labor. The pushing effort should be reserved for the second stage. To help the woman refrain from pushing, the attendant may introduce various breathing techniques (such as panting), changes of position, backrubs, foot massages, empathic conversation, and encouragement and reassurance about the progress and normality of labor. The attendant should also reassure the woman that sensations stemming from descent of the fetal head and uterine action are normal and should not be resisted.

Labor Support at Difficult Moments

If the mother is experiencing a great deal of pain or exhaustion, with consequent loss of morale and/or effectiveness of contractions, the following approaches may be helpful:

- Give her intense labor support, every minute of every contraction and in between. Give her almost constant eye contact and physical support.

- Leave her totally alone for a brief period so that she can attend to her own sensations and find out what is happening subjectively for her. Sometimes the mother and father will work things out if left alone for a while.

- Change the environment for her.

- Change her physical condition or her sensations. Have her push fluids, walk up and down stairs to loosen up, or deep squat to widen the pelvis and increase her pelvic sensations.

- Plant hypnotic suggestion. Speak quietly in her ear and tell her what you want to happen. Repeat key words like "open," "move down," "melt," "let go," "contract." However, a pep talk that sounds like a broken record will just be irritating.

- Focus her attention on the baby. Remind her that the baby really is coming. Get her to imagine the baby and to visualize how her body is working to support the baby (breathing gives the baby oxygen, resting gives the baby rest). Do not make it sound like a contest between her and the baby. Stress that they are working in harmony.

- Communicate confidence in her progress and in her ability to labor successfully, despite momentary loss of "control." If the family is unfamiliar with the intensity of normal labor, it will be the attendant's job to remind the woman and her partner of their deeper intentions and long-range goals and to inspire them to go on. The attendant may have to assume an authoritative stance, trying to keep everyone calm and if necessary asking unsupportive or anxious people to leave.

- Be aware of her emotional vulnerability and the background of intense sensation against which she hears what is said to her. Many women report a combination of highly focused self-awareness and selective attention to what people say and do during labor. The potential for distortion in this mode of perception makes it important to speak at close enough range and at sufficient volume for the woman to hear, to time communications appropriately (e.g., not at the height of a contraction), and to be aware of the possibility of misinterpretation. Half-heard remarks or laughter may be misconstrued by a woman who is anxious about her performance. On the other hand, reassurance about the progress of the labor with *genuine* encouragement and praise can be very effective, especially in the context of a trusting relationship established during the pregnancy.

Both the mother and baby must be carefully monitored during periods of increased stress. Before intervening in a woman's labor the attendant must make sure that she really needs help. A heavy-handed approach at home is just as undermining as an unnecessary medical intervention in the hospital. Each labor is different. What should or should not be done can only be discerned by close personal attention to the individual woman.

When it is necessary to report on progress or raise the question of abnormalities, some attention must be given to the timing of the communication and to the ways in which it may be, and ultimately is, received. In attempting to maximize the receptivity of the laboring woman and her partner, it may be useful for the two attendants first to discuss what is to be said and how it will be said, so as to anticipate the questions and concerns that may arise. Such a rehearsal often serves to clarify diagnostic perceptions and expand therapeutic options. Members of the attending team should feel free to be critical devil's advocates and not be inhibited about whatever suggestions, ideas, or criticisms they have, as long as they discuss these disagreements privately rather than argue in front of the family. The different options can be presented to the family, but only after the attendants have "agreed to disagree."

SECOND STAGE

The second stage begins with full dilatation and ends with the birth of the baby. Most of the descent of the baby takes place immediately prior to and during the second stage.

Guidelines for Monitoring

Screening for second-stage problems includes continued observation of both mother and baby. The baby's heart should be listened to after every or perhaps (if mild) every other contraction. Occasionally the fetal heart tones should be listened to through a contraction, as in the first stage. The closer together the contractions and the less advantageous a position the mother is in for blood flow to the baby (see discussion of positions for delivery in this chapter), the more the baby should be followed. The fetal heart will move lower and rotate toward the midline as the baby descends. If the heart tones cannot be heard because the baby's back is moving under the pubic bone, an ultrasound monitor can usually detect them.

In monitoring the mother's condition, the attendant must keep in mind that blood pressure and pulse normally increase in the second stage. The mother should still move around as much as possible and continue to empty her bladder.

Vaginal examinations should be performed if one needs more information about descent. If the mother suddenly says, "The baby's coming!" and her rectum starts to open up, a vaginal examination is probably unnecessary. Conversely, if a woman has been pushing for half an hour to an hour with no apparent change, a vaginal examination will give both the attendant and the mother useful information.

Using a sterile glove and ample lubrication, the attendant should check for (1) descent of fetal head in relation to the ischial spines (station), (2) lip of cervix, (3) position of the baby's head, (4) progress of internal rotation, (5) fetal scalp color[24], and (6) degree of moulding and caput formation. The attendant's hand should be left in during a contraction to feel for descent during the contraction. If there is any delay, often the attendant can give a few suggestions, push up a persistent lip of cervix (if this can be easily and gently done), or tell the woman when her push is effective. Firm intravaginal pressure directed posteriorly toward the rectum can be applied to diminish soft tissue resistance to fetal descent and possibly stimulate uterine contractions and the bearing down reflex.

Labor Support

Labor support in the second stage is similar to that in the first stage. As full dilatation is achieved, the woman should have the opportunity to enjoy any lull in her labor before the urge to push is felt. It is not good practice to coach women to push as forcefully as possible during contractions in the second stage. There are wide variations in women's perceptions of the need to push, and for the most part these perceptions are reliable indicators of what is helpful in encouraging descent. Maternal efforts are not only more effective, but safer for the baby when they are spontaneous and unforced.[25] A woman should be encouraged to push when, how, and as long as she wishes unless there is a particular problem.

Some women may need to be encouraged to push. Some are inhibited from pushing after having just spent hours refraining from doing so. Others are inhibited by fears about birth and unfamiliarity with the sensations that may accompany descent (back pain and rectal pressure followed by feelings of imminent tearing or burning). On the other hand, although some women find the second stage more painful than the first, others experience a sense of well-being and of voluntary participation accompanied by progress, which by contrast with the first stage comes as a relief.

Frequently a mother will ask what to do, not because she cannot push, but because she feels momentarily overwhelmed by feelings of strangeness and feared loss of control. The attendant should take the time to cue her back into her own sensations rather than tell her how to push. She can deep breathe, try to relax, walk around, or squat and wait until the body's intention is irresistible. When she starts to give in to the sensation, she should be encouraged with words like "yes," "that's it," or "good" rather than "push into your bottom" or "hold your breath" or other specific directions that may confuse her. She should be encouraged to "release" her baby rather than "push" it out. She should not be trying to ram her baby out against a tense pelvic floor. When she can be felt to relax, she should be given positive feedback that she is stretching just as she should be.

In the absence of fetal distress or arrest of descent, a second stage conducted in harmony with the rhythms of the woman's body need have no arbitrary time limit. (See discussion of prolonged labor under "complications of labor." The family should be informed that this point of view is at variance with standard obstetric practice.) Caldeyro-Barcia[26] found no difference in Apgar scores or blood gas values with second stages of 15 minutes versus three hours or more. A woman who flows with the contractions, rather than forcing them, is calmer and more aware for crowning, so that there is less likelihood of tearing and less need for an episiotomy. Hurrying the second stage, on the other hand, may not give the pelvic floor sufficient time to distend.

Still, it is also not good practice to let a woman flounder around indefinitely if no progress is being made. If the woman cannot organize her pushing efforts after an hour with no progress, more specific directions may need to be given. During a vaginal examination, the attendant should help her get synchronized with her uterus by telling her when the baby's head is felt to descend with the peak of the contraction. Again, pressing down (quite firmly) over the rectum from the vagina will help increase her urge.

The mother should not be forced into any particular position. Careful observation of her mood, body tension, and so forth (i.e., of the whole woman) will show where she needs support and when she needs a change. Since she will continue to need to urinate, going to the bathroom is still a good device for bringing about a change of scene. Often the toilet is a very effective place to push.

As soon as any part of the head is visible, others will want to see it. Children enjoy seeing the baby's hair. The first view of the baby often energizes everyone, no matter how tired. Since the mother may need some energy, too, she should be given a mirror and encouraged to touch the head as soon as she can. This visualization and hands-on experience of the birth can allow the woman to regain control and be drawn back into the miracle of birth. Visual and tactile contact with the descending baby also serves as a reminder of the whole point of the birth process. This physical affirmation of the choice of becoming a parent can return the woman to a sense of human purposefulness in creating a new family member.

Preparation for Delivery

When delivery is imminent, the mother will need to be supported by her family (and by a second attendant if there is one) while the attendant finishes setting up the equipment for delivery. Often an apprentice or assistant can do the setting up.

1. Prepare the oxygen tank for use and attach tubing. See that the DeLee suction catheter is at hand, as well as any other equipment for resuscitation. Avoid leaving things where they may make people trip.
2. Open the birth kit. Emergency supplies should be accessible but need not be laid out all over the room.
3. A crock pot or electric skillet with warm water or camomile tea for compresses should be plugged in near the delivery area.
4. Immediate supplies for the normal birth should be on a tray next to the attendant. These should include receiving blankets, bulb syringe, and cord tying instruments. Also handy should be sterile gloves, perineal oil for massage, sterile 4 × 4 gauze pads, flashlight, and mirror. The receiving blankets can be warmed by a heating pad on the highest setting or placed on a warm radiator.

Before the delivery, the social environment is reassessed. It is important that all attendants are comfortable and that the atmosphere is quiet and warm enough for the baby.

Positions for Delivery

The following positions can be used for delivery. Ideally, the mother should determine the position that is best for her, and the attendant should be prepared to assist her in that position.

Lithotomy Position

The lithotomy position is not recommended for any reason. Compression of the vena cava and the aorta by the uterus may interfere with blood flow to and from the uterus and fetoplacental unit. The lithotomy position also entails maternal effort against gravity, since the baby is pushed uphill through the pelvic outlet.[27]

Lamaze Position

Advantages. The Lamaze position (semi-sit, dorsal) makes good use of gravity. There is good visibility for the mother and others present, and access to fetal heart tones is good, although fetal circulation may be slightly compromised.

Disadvantages. The attendant's access to the perineum is poor, and the mobility of the coccyx may be impaired. (The mother's bottom can be lifted up on a bolster or padded overturned drawer or stack of folded towels, or she can be brought to the edge of the bed or sofa and people can support her legs.) This position puts more stress on the perineum than some positions but less than that of the lithotomy position. The more relaxed the legs, the more relaxed is the perineum. (This is true for all positions.)

Side Lying

Advantages. In the side lying (lateral, Sims) position fetal oxygenation is good, and access to fetal heart tones is good if the mother is lying on the opposite side from the baby's back. Access to the perineum is excellent, especially if the attendant sits around behind the mother's legs. The father can coach and support his partner *and* catch the baby.

Disadvantages. Access to fetal heart tones is poor if the mother is lying on the same side as the baby's back. The effect of gravity is almost nonexistent. (This may be desirable when (as with a multipara with a small baby) there is a need to slow down and thereby reduce the force of the final descent, both to protect the mother against tearing and to minimize sudden pressure on the baby's head.) The weight of the mother's upper leg must be entirely supported by others, either by having someone hold it or by having the mother put her foot on the attendant's or someone else's shoulder. The mother may experience back pain (good alignment with strong back support and leg support under the knee must be maintained). The mother may feel too passive if she is lying too far down. If so, she can sit up more while remaining in a lateral position. The attendant stands or sits behind the woman, controlling the perineum with one hand and the descent and flexion of the baby's head with the other hand from around the top of the upper leg over the mother's abdomen.

Hands and Knees

Advantages. The hands and knees (kneeling and leaning on pillows) position is excellent for fetal oxygenation. It is good for maternal control, good for access to the perineum, and good for pelvic movement. It is also easy to apply pressure to the back, good for rotating posterior positions and breech deliveries, good for suctioning the baby if necessary, and good for shoulder dystocia.

Disadvantages. If this position is used it is hard to maintain eye contact with the mother, and hard (but not impossible) for the mother to see or feel baby's head. It can be disorienting to the inexperienced practitioner, and it is hard to hear fetal heart tones (a fetoscope with long tubing or ultrasound monitor can be used between the mother's legs from behind). The baby can get a noseful of hindwaters, and it is hard for the mother to catch the baby (have someone support her shoulders from the front; then, as the baby's shoulders are born, aim the baby up toward mother's abdomen so that she can reach down and catch it). This position is poor if there is a tight nuchal cord because it does not allow access to the back of the baby's head, where the cord must be cut.

Standing

Advantages. Standing (perhaps supported by a person or a wall or railing) is excellent for fetal oxygenation and access to the perineum and allows great freedom of movement. There may be a reduced risk of perineal tears (undocumented). The father can help the mother catch the baby from in front while an assistant monitors fetal heart tones from in front and the attendant monitors the perineum from behind.

Disadvantages. The mother may not feel strong enough to stand up on her own. Delivery can occur too quickly if the mother is not attentive to her sensations or not receptive to coaching.

Squatting

Advantages. Squatting (hanging or supported) is excellent for access to the perineum and circulation. Pelvic diameters are maximized[28] and there may be a reduced risk of perineal tears (undocumented). As shown by Odent,[29] the mother can hang on rope attached to rafters or other support or can be held by the axillae from behind by the male partner or friend who leans back with straight arms to bear her weight as she squats low enough for relaxed legs to be flexed. These upright positions may improve a poor fetal heart tone pattern that is not improved by lying on the side.

Disadvantages. The position is hard on the knees unless the woman has good support. It prevents her from catching the baby.

Perineal Care at Delivery

Episiotomy

Although comparative data on the advantages and disadvantages of episiotomy have not been obtained for large study groups over long periods of time, the experience of the authors and other practitioners indicates that the preparation of the perineum with massage and hot compresses is as effective as episiotomy in minimizing both short-term damage (i.e., perineal tears, especially those with extension to the rectum or bladder) and long-term damage (i.e., cystoceles, rectoceles, relaxation of uterine supports). Prophylactic episiotomies to preserve the integrity of the pelvic floor are, therefore, not recommended.

Episiotomy in home births should be reserved for conditions such as the following:

- arrest in progress by resistant perineum with thick or heavily muscled nondistensible soft tissue
- imminent threat of laceration anticipated by inspection of the perineum during bearing-down efforts
- fetal distress requiring rapid delivery. Episiotomy may also allow for corrective manipulation of the baby's position or the application of a vacuum extractor.

Even under these circumstances, an episiotomy can often be avoided by squatting or other changes in position.

The timing of the episiotomy is important. Performed too late, the procedure will fail to prevent lacerations and protect the pelvic floor. Made too soon, the incision will lead to excessive loss of blood. Episiotomy should be made when the perineum is bulging, when 3 to 4 cm of skull is visible during contraction, and when the presenting part can be delivered within the next three to five contractions.

Perineal Massage

The need for perineal massage will have been assessed during previous examinations. The woman's obstetric history is also a useful indicator. If her other children were born over intact perineums, this one probably will be, too. How much massage is needed will be determined as it is being done.

As the head becomes visible at the outlet, gentle massage is started. Liberal amounts of oil are used; the hymenal ring is found and massaged back and forth slowly while the tissues are stretched and assessed. The woman is asked how it feels. If she likes it, then it is continued; if she does not, only as much as seems clinically necessary is done. The motion is circled up to the pubic arch on either side.

Externally the entire vulva can be massaged, with emphasis on the band of the perineal body stretched across and the tighter skin of the fourchette.

Massage is less easy in the more upright positions. Fortunately, it is also probably less important, since the stress on the perineum is reduced.

Hot Compresses

Heat to the perineum serves three purposes: (1) it helps improve circulation in the perineal tissues, (2) it helps the mother relax her pelvic and rectal areas, and (3) it gives her pleasure when she is feeling somewhat uncomfortable everywhere else.

Warm washcloths hold heat well but cannot be reused if fecal material gets on them. Thick gauze pads can easily be discarded but do not hold heat well. Too much heat to the perineum may cause excessive congestion in the tissues and increase rather than decrease the chance of tearing. Ice can be useful in reducing a swollen perineum and often feels good as well.

The Delivery

Rupture of the Membranes

The membranes should not be ruptured until the last possible moment. The attendant will have to decide when to rupture the membranes if they have not ruptured spontaneously at full dilatation and there appears to be nothing else keeping the baby from being born. If the baby is born in the membranes, they will have to be opened and stripped off the baby's face as it is born. "Old midwives' tales" have it that if a baby girl is "born in the caul" she is destined to become a midwife. If a boy is born in the caul and becomes a sailor he will never drown.

Birth of the Head

When the mother is in the dorsal or lateral position, the perineum has a tendency to be swept downward and forward as the head begins to extend. This puts the thinned perineum directly in the way of the continued descent of the head and increases the possibility of tearing. To counteract this tendency two maneuvers are helpful. One is to keep the head flexed as long as possible. The second is to keep the perineum stretched backward and upward close to the ischial tuberosities. The sooner the head passes through the vulval ring in its descent, the less thinned the perineum will have to be.

To keep the head flexed, the perineal hand is used to press gently on the baby's lower face through the perineum and the other hand pushes downward and backward on the occiput. Once the entire occiput has come under the symphysis, extension of the head is no longer a stress on the perineum because the biparietal diameter is almost through the vulval ring. Gentle extension will now deliver the face slowly (sometimes even between contractions), centimeter by centimeter—eyebrows, eyes, nose, upper lip, and finally chin. Holding the vertex in one hand and the perineum in the other, the attendant slowly separates the two hands during a contraction or lets the uterus do it (with no maternal pushing) during a contraction, while making sure that the extension is not too rapid. The woman may need to be reminded to pant or blow in order to avoid voluntary expulsive efforts. Eye contact (when possible) and clear and repeated verbal directions may be necessary.

In the more upright positions (standing, squatting, or kneeling) the perineum will tend to retract more on its own and the head will stay in flexion longer. Much less maneuvering (if any) is necessary to achieve a tear-free delivery. Any mucus—or oil used in perineal massage—is wiped off the baby's face with a sterile gauze pad.

Nuchal Cord

Once the chin is delivered, a thorough check for a cord around the neck or shoulders is made. The loop is pulled down and over the baby's head if possible. If the loop does not quite fit over the head, it is left and slipped over the shoulders as they are born. If the cord is too tight, it is clamped in two places and cut between the clamps, and the two segments are unwound. The baby is delivered quickly and the attendant must be prepared to resuscitate.

Delivery of the Shoulders

The baby's head will rotate to the transverse position as the shoulders move into the anteroposterior diameter. When the shoulders start to come with the next contraction, the parents can be told to reach down to the baby if they want to catch it.

If there is any delay in the anterior shoulder coming under the symphysis, gentle traction on the baby's head toward the mother's rectum will bring the anterior shoulder barely into view. As the shoulders come out, the head should then be guided back up toward the mother and/or father (with an eye on the posterior shoulder as it sweeps the perineum). One hand can guard the perineum if necessary. If there is a nuchal arm, all that need be done is to guard the perineum carefully to prevent a tear in case the elbow pops out. Sometimes more complex assisted tractions and rotations of the shoulder are required. (See discussion of shoulder dystocia later in this chapter.) All manipulations of the baby should be done with extreme gentleness.

Aftermath

If the parents do not reach down and catch the baby, the baby's head and body are guided upward (following the curve of Carus formed by the passageway through the pelvis and vagina[30]) and over the pubic bone onto the mother's abdomen. The baby is placed sideways with the head slightly dependent, if possible, to drain any mucus and covered quickly with a warm blanket.

The parents can be asked about the sex of the baby if they do not discover it spontaneously (as is sometimes the case when the mother catches the baby and places it immediately on her abdomen). The need for suctioning is quickly assessed and a one-minute Apgar score is done (see Chapter 12). The baby's pulse can be felt over the sternum with two fingers. Color is checked for with a flashlight if it is dark.

The timing of cord clamping is a controversial issue. The authors' practice is to delay clamping of the cord until pulsation ceases. As much as 100 milliliters of blood may be shifted from the placenta to the infant before cord clamping takes place, particularly with the infant in a dependent position in relation to the placenta (with gravity assisting this transfer and respiratory efforts adding to the negative pressure drawing blood through the umbilical vessels). Immediate clamping of the cord or elevation of the baby above the level of the placenta may prevent this placentofetal transfusion or reverse its direction. Immediate clamping of the cord with Rh negative women should be considered if there is any significant risk of sensitization having occurred (as evidenced by titers performed during pregnancy, amniotic fluid studies, and/or failure to use rhoGAM prophylactically at the 28th week).

Pulsation usually stops within five minutes after the birth. At that time the cord should be clamped or tied (with a square knot) about 1½ inches from the baby's abdomen. The cord is held away from the baby and then a hemostat is placed an inch away from the first tie. The father, mother, or a sibling can then cut the cord if they desire. A gauze pad may be placed under the area to be cut to keep any blood off the baby. Cord ties or shoelaces should be trimmed to avoid their getting tangled in the receiving blankets or elsewhere.

The rest of the cord is placed between the mother's legs where it will not be pulled accidentally, and the hemostat is removed temporarily to allow blood to drain into the placenta bowl. The blankets are replaced if they are wet, making sure to keep the baby's head covered. (Some home birth supply houses sell cotton knit caps for this purpose.) Then the attendant can step back and let the parents enjoy the baby. While they are doing this a five-minute Apgar score should be done as unobtrusively as possible.

The attendant must remain conscious of the extraordinary importance of the initial contact between the parents and their baby. A balance should be reached between the often enlivening and catalytic effect of having the parents observe the experienced birth attendant, who can handle a baby with greater assurance and is more attuned to the early behaviors of the newborn, and the parents' need to exercise their own innate capacity to bond with their child. The attendants must also strike a balance between continuing clinical evaluation in the third stage and the creation of a positive atmosphere for family bonding. Toward these ends, there is a natural division of labor in which one attendant assists the parents with bonding and early care of the newborn while the other attends to the management of the third stage. For the first attendant all that is necessary is to monitor the newborn for any pathological signs of distress and, if necessary, to give the parents an occasional word of encouragement or reassurance, reminders about protecting the baby from heat loss or excessive neck motion, and instruction in breast-feeding.

The mother is encouraged to put the baby to breast. The more upright she is sitting, the easier it will be for the baby to get the nipple. (A supportive upright position, together with verbal stimulation, also facilitates eye-to-eye contact.) The mother is assisted in compressing her areola if necessary and shown how the baby roots.

Now is the time to institute good nursing habits and optimal nursing techniques. Use of the belly to belly position is encouraged. The mother and baby are exactly front to front so that the baby does not have to keep its head turned to the side to nurse (once it has latched on). As much of the mother's nipple is in the baby's mouth as possible. The baby will have to open its mouth wide and keep its tongue under the breast.

Everyone can be encouraged to touch and enjoy the baby, to praise the mother, and to express their emotions. However, the party should not begin in earnest until the placenta is out. The mother is asked if she has any cramps or contractions. If convenient, an attendant can leave a hand on her fundus (without "fiddling," i.e., massaging or stimulating it) to check for contractions.

Further guidelines on newborn care can be found in Chapter 12.

THIRD STAGE

The following signs of placental separation must be looked for:

- gush of blood from the vagina
- lengthening of visible cord
- change in size and shape of the uterus (globular shape, firm consistency) with perception of a contraction

If these signs are equivocal or absent, another method of assessing placental separation is cephalad fundal pressure. The cord will move upward in the case of an unseparated placenta (or, more rarely, a placenta that is trapped in the cervical canal) but will be relatively unaffected by the movement if the placenta has separated.

The attendant must not pull on the cord to determine if separation has occurred. Even when it is necessary to "guard" the fundus (i.e., keep a hand in to feel for changes in shape), it is important not to "fiddle" with (i.e., rub or poke) it. Interference during the third stage of labor, either by pulling on the cord or by attempting an active expression of the placenta before separation has occurred, probably represents the greatest hazard to a mother in a home birth, in that it significantly increases the risk of postpartum hemorrhage or inversion of the uterus. Protocols for management of postpartum hemorrhage and failure of placental separation or expulsion can be found in the discussion of complications of labor in a later section of this chapter. These should be consulted if the placenta is not spontaneously delivered within 20 minutes after the birth of the baby and especially if it is not delivered within 45 minutes.

When the signs of placental separation are observed and a contraction is felt by the mother or attendant (while "guarding"), the placenta generally is ready for expulsion. The attendant assists the mother as she squats over the placenta bowl and bears down. The mother may be able to handle the baby herself or she may need to hand it to someone else. If she seems too distracted by the baby to concentrate, the attendant should gently remind her of what needs to be done and then wait until she is ready. Controlled cord traction is sometimes necessary to complete the third stage while minimizing the mother's active participation so that she can concentrate on bonding with the baby.

A squatting position between separation and expulsion of the placenta is believed to aid in expulsion and reduce blood loss, although these advantages are undocumented. In addition to the mechanical benefits of the squatting position, the uterus tends to fall forward away from the inferior vena cava, thus reducing the chance of excessive bleeding from the tourniquet effect on the vena cava that would occur in the supine position. However, if the mother feels uncomfortable when squatting, she should sit down.

As the placenta emerges the membranes may need to be teased or twisted out gently between the attendant's fingers to try to avoid leaving pieces of membrane behind. It often helps for the woman to cough. When the placenta has been expelled, the uterus should be checked to confirm that it is contracted. The placenta, membranes, and cord should be inspected for completeness. The presence of placental abnormalities such as infarcts, calcifications, absent cotyledons, or areas of tearing that might indicate a retained portion of the placenta or membranes in the uterus should be assessed. The cord should have three blood vessels; deviations from this norm can be associated with congenital abnormalities.

FOURTH STAGE

The fourth stage is defined as lasting one hour after the delivery of the placenta. The birth attendant should remain in the home a minimum of two hours after the birth. During this time there should be a few minutes for the attendant to sit down and enjoy the scene. However, there are also continuing clinical responsibilities with regard to both the mother and the baby.

In addition to examining the mother's vagina for tears, the attendant should observe the mother in a more global way until she is stable (i.e., is moving comfortably in bed, has stable vital signs, and has had something to eat and drink). The mother should also urinate. She can take a shower if she feels well. Someone should be in the shower with her in case she faints or bleeds, and someone should be nearby to support her, if necessary, when she walks. While she is in the shower the bed should be changed and the birth room cleaned up. If the mother remains in bed she should urinate in a pot or bedpan (if available) and should be given a partial bed bath. She may want to put on a clean nightgown and sanitary pad. If the perineum is sore or swollen, ice compresses may be soothing. A sterile glove is filled with crushed ice, tied like a balloon, wrapped in a sterile gauze pad, and placed between the perineum and the sanitary pad. If stitches are necessary, sometimes it may be easier to reduce the swelling before starting to suture. Except in an emergency the parents should have some time together with the baby before a procedure such as suturing is begun.

The baby's condition also requires further monitoring. Occasionally, babies who are well at 15 minutes are not well at 45 minutes. (See Chapter 12 for problematic conditions in the newborn.) The father, siblings, and significant others should have their turn with the baby.

Before leaving the home, the attendant should see that the baby has nursed successfully. The attendant also performs the newborn examination (see Chapter 12), teaches the mother how to feel her uterus, and gives the family postpartum instructions (see Chapter 13).

COMPLICATIONS OF LABOR

This chapter has thus far described normal labor and delivery in properly screened, prepared, and attended home births. Although the attendant can expect most such births to go smoothly, the recognition and management of complications is nonetheless an essential part of the attendant's job. The remainder of this chapter outlines the major complications of labor that the birth attendant working in the home must be prepared to face. A timely, effective, and discriminating response to these complications when they occur can be crucial to the well-being of the mother and baby.

Prolonged Labor

Prolonged labor is the most common complication of labor. Together with the arrest disorders, it is also the most controversial. Prolonged labors will constitute the bulk of transfers from a home birth service, especially one that includes primigravidas. Yet the range of transfer rates in such services[31] suggests that there are considerable variations in the diagnosis and treatment of prolonged as well as arrested labors.

Whether a home birth can be successfully completed after a labor pattern deviating from the standard develops is affected both directly and indirectly by the attendant's viewpoint concerning the implications of a "failure to progress"—directly in terms of the attendant's policy and clinical judgments, indirectly in that the attendant's attitude itself influences the woman's ability to progress. A new practitioner is justified in being conservative (i.e., erring on the side of more transfers). As one gains experience, one's intuition and clinical judgment become more finely tuned. One becomes better able to get to the root of a labor problem and help the parents out of it rather than transfer the woman to a hospital.[32] This is not to say that there are no objective parameters that are useful in dealing with problematic labors. However, it is commonly observed that transfers (or augmentations or cesareans) occur not always at an objective point in the clinical course but often when the practitioner has a feeling of hopelessness. What laboring woman has the strength to go on when her attendant has given up?

It is generally acknowledged that medical interventions such as early artificial rupture of membranes or oxytocin augmentation have *no* place in labors at home. That still leaves many safer techniques for stimulating labor, which will be discussed here.

If a transfer is finally required, the attendant should not prepare the family for surgical delivery unless there is an emergency, such as a pathological retraction ring or fetal distress. Disappointment over leaving home coupled with fear of a probable cesarean section can make it very difficult for a woman to continue in her labor. The parents instead should be encouraged to think of the hospital as a source of help and hope (see Chapters 6 and 7).

The Friedman Curve

Some clinicians use the Friedman curve[33] (with which labor is analyzed by plotting descent and dilatation over time) and the clinical recommendations associated with it to guide their diagnosis and management of abnormal labor patterns. Others find the curve useful as a conceptual model but do not adhere strictly to Friedman's management guidelines.

According to Friedman, there are three distinct time periods in the process of dilatation and descent, as shown in Table 11-1. The *preparatory* division of labor is that period in which the cervix is being prepared for later dilatation. During this division the myometrial contractility of the uterus becomes organized and the cervix fully "ripened." Second, the

Table 11-1 Principal Clinical Features of the Functional Divisions of Labor

Characteristic	Preparatory division	Dilatational division	Pelvic division
Functions	Contractions coordinated, polarized, oriented; cervix prepared	Cervix actively dilated	Pelvis negotiated; mechanisms of labor; fetal descent; delivery
Interval	Latent and acceleration phases	Phase of maximum slope	Deceleration phase and second stage
Measurement	Elapsed duration	Linear rate of dilatation	Linear rate of descent
Diagnosable disorders	Prolonged latent phase	Protracted dilatation; protracted descent	Prolonged deceleration; secondary arrest of dilatation; arrest of descent; failure of descent

Source: Reprinted from *Labor: Clinical Evaluation and Management,* 2nd ed., by Emanuel A. Friedman, with permission of Appleton-Century-Crofts, © 1978.

---

relatively brief interval in which almost all cervical dilatation occurs constitutes the so-called *dilatational* division. Third, there is the deceleration of dilatation and the second-stage descent in its entirety. It is in this *pelvic* division of labor that the greatest part of descent and all other fetal mechanisms of labor take place.

The divisions of labor are further subdivided into phases. The latent phase of the first stage is timed from the onset of contractions to dilatation of about 3 cm. (If the contractions stop, suggesting false labor, timing stops and starts over again when the contractions resume.) This phase, which corresponds to the preparatory division of labor, is characterized as prolonged when it exceeds 20 hours in the primigravida or 14 hours in the multipara[34] A prolonged latent phase is not diagnostic of any other problem and in and of itself poses no threat to the mother or the baby. If the mother and the baby are in good condition, one can wait for the active phase. If intervention seems wise, labor can either be stopped or stimulated as described below.

The active phase of labor in the first stage begins at 3 to 4 cm and lasts until full dilatation. There is a period of acceleration when contractions begin to get stronger, followed by a brief period of very strong contractions and rapid dilatation called the phase of maximal slope. As full dilatation is reached (8 to10 cm) the progress slows down slightly, signifying the so-called deceleration phase. Prolonged or protracted active phase can occur in any of these three periods. It may be related to poor quality contractions, to the woman's reaction to the contractions or to a less than optimal fetopelvic relationship, including occiput posterior position, face or brow presentation, or (more rarely) cephalopelvic disproportion. The upper limit of normal active phase as defined by Friedman is 12 hours for a primigravida and 6 hours for a multipara.[35]

Prolonged labor in second stage is defined as over 2 hours in the primigravida and 1 hour in the multigravida.[36]

In the authors' practice prolonged labor at any stage is not considered reason for intervention so long as some progress is being made and no other difficulties are noted. Careful attention to both the mother's and the baby's condition is essential. Therapeutic efforts to stop or stimulate labor are described in the following section.

Arrested Labor

The arrest disorders constitute the more serious (and more controversial) category of abnormal labor patterns. These problems include arrest of dilatation in any part of active phase and arrest of descent in second stage. Both can occur simultaneously during the deceleration phase when dilatation and descent both normally occur. They can further complicate prolonged labor in the active phase of first stage or in second stage.

Diagnostic Criteria

In the face of arrested labor at any point, the attendant should take into account the following diagnostic factors. Much of the information specified will be apparent to an attendant who has been in the home throughout the labor.

Character of Contractions. Relevant data about the contractions include the basic information about interval, duration, and intensity. Are the contractions appropriate for the dilatation? Do the contractions appear to have a normal gradient pattern, or can a dysfunctional action be identified?[37] Are there any contractions at all? Are there such intense contractions that the lower segment is thinning dangerously and therefore is at risk of rupture?

If there are no contractions, the woman either is no longer in labor or, if the cervix did not dilate, was in false labor. If there are hypotonic, hypertonic, or other inefficient contractions, they should be stopped or stimulated according to the situation (see Table 11-2 and Figure 11-1). If there is a pathological retraction ring (Bandl's ring) or any suspicion that the lower segment is thinning owing to intense contractions and an unresponsive cervix, transfer should occur immediately to anticipate being able to manage uterine rupture. If the arrest of progress occurs during what is already a prolonged labor, a consultant should be called and transfer considered.

Condition of Mother. The condition of the mother can best be evaluated by the person who has been labor-sitting with her. Both her physical and emotional state are relevant. Is she exhausted (which may inhibit uterine action), demoralized, afraid (of what?), in pain (where?), dehydrated, ketotic, unsupported by family and friends, or under any other kind of stress? If she is in good condition in all these respects, the attendant may decide to wait and try other remedies before transferring. If she is physically normal by objective measures but upset or afraid, one can try to help her face the problem and move through it. For example, sometimes women who become afraid of the sensations of descent can actually hold up their labor. A sensitive inquiry and a gentle but firm educational vaginal examination can help a woman resume her progress in labor. If in fact the woman's physical condition is just beginning to deteriorate, it may be reversed by appropriate intervention such as rehydrating her and giving her honey or some other concentrated sweet food for calories. On the other hand, a mother in intractable pain, who is out of control despite the best efforts of those who know and love her best, probably will not dilate until she gets some more potent pain relief through anesthetic or analgesic drugs, which should be given only in the hospital.

Condition of Baby. The condition of the baby must be inferred from the other three factors listed here and from any possible indications of fetal distress. (See the following section.) Clearly, any indication of fetal distress with an arrest of labor requires immediate transport.

Possibility of Cephalopelvic Disproportion. The possibility of cephalopelvic disproportion (CPD) is frequently linked in clinicians' minds with arrest of progress. If an arrest occurs and the clinician believes that this particular baby could not possibly fit through this particular pelvis, transfer is the only appropriate reaction to what amounts to a failed trial of labor.

Unfortunately, the diagnosis of CPD, especially in the home, is quite problematic. It has repeatedly been demonstrated that pelvimetry is not useful in predicting successful vaginal delivery.[38] And yet using the labor pattern as diagnostic (or suspicious) of CPD is also questionable and can lead to a self-fulfilling prophecy for the attendant and thereby for the laboring woman as she senses the attendant "going through the motions" of attempting a vaginal birth.

At best one can identify when one is dealing with a "tight fit." Indications that greater than usual accommodations will need to be made for the baby to descend include the following:

- posterior presentations—may either deliver posterior or take the extra time to rotate; presenting diameter is larger and fits less well to shape of pelvis; moulding is less effective.
- deflexed head—may need stronger contractions to flex it enough to descend well or may descend slowly while remaining deflexed, thereby presenting a larger diameter
- extreme caput formation—indicates increased pressure on fetal head; actual descent may or may not be occurring.
- extreme moulding—characterized by overlapping sutures (usually parietal over occipital and one parietal over the other at the sagittal suture). Is biparietal diameter descending or is apparent descent just moulding?
- edema of cervix—previously effaced cervix getting thicker and appearing to be closing down
- edema of vulva—occurs when mother is pushing hard without bringing about much fetal descent
- head compression fetal heart tone pattern (see following section on fetal distress)
- high station of head despite good contractions; the cervix sometimes hangs "like an empty sleeve" with fetal head not applied to it.
- clinically evident small pelvic dimensions such as narrow inlet, mid-pelvis, or outlet

None of these signs is in itself diagnostic of disproportion. However, they should alert the clinician to the reason for the slow progress. They are also considerations in making a prognosis with a tight fit.

Family's Wishes and Values. Taking all signs together, the clinician should decide if normal vaginal delivery in the home is likely, in question but possible, highly unlikely but not impossible, or impossible or dangerous. The family's intuitions, feelings, and values should also be considered. The decision about how much they are willing to endure may be ultimately theirs, although society and health care providers also have pertinent values and interests to protect (see Chapter 4).

Therapeutic Options

The standard obstetric protocols for management of arrested as well as prolonged labor are presented in Table 11-2 and Figure 11-1. The tables exemplify the descriptive usefulness of Friedman's diagnostic categories even for clinicians who dissent from some of his recommendations. Home birth attendants should know about the standard hospital procedures in order both to obtain informed consent for other clinical strategies in the home and to provide knowledgeable support for families following transfer to hospital for measures such as cesarean section. Nonetheless, the differences in approach are worth noting. In the authors' practice, oxytocin is not used to stimulate labor in the home. Furthermore, it is the widely shared (albeit undocumented and anecdotal) experience of midwives that

Table 11-2 Patterns of Dysfunctional Labor

	Prolonged latent phase	Protraction disorders	Arrest disorders
Diagnosis	Nulliparas > 20 hr Multiparas > 14 hr	*Dilatation* Nulliparas < 1.2 cm/hr Multiparas < 1.5 cm/hr *Descent* Nulliparas < 1.0 cm/hr Multiparas < 2.0 cm/hr	*Deceleration* Nulliparas > 3 hr Multiparas > 1 hr *Dilation* Arrest > 2 hr *Descent* Arrest > 1 hr
Etiology	Excess sedation Unprepared cervix False labor Anesthesia Uterine dysfunction	Unknown CPD 28% Malposition Excess sedation Anesthesia	CPD 45% Malposition Excess sedation Anesthesia
Therapy	*Rest*	*Support* Avoid inhibition	*Cesarean* for CPD *Oxytocin* if no CPD
Response	85% "cure" 10% out of labor	90% progress	94% "cure"
Delivery	Vaginal	Vaginal Cesarean for CPD	Cesarean for CPD Vaginal (by response)
Fetal risk	Not increased	Slightly increased	Threefold increase

CPD, cephalopelvic disproportion.

Source: Reprinted from "Disordered Labor: Objective Evaluation and Management," by Emanuel A. Friedman, *Journal of Family Practice,* vol. 2, p. 170, with permission of Appleton-Century-Crofts, © 1975.

Figure 11-1 Summary of Friedman's Recommendations for
Management of Dysfunctional Patterns of Labor

	Preferred Treatment	*Exceptionally*
Prolonged Latent Phase	Therapeutic Rest	Oxytocin for exigencies
Protraction Disorders	Expectancy and Support	Cesarean Section for CPD
Arrest Disorders — *With CPD*	Cesarean Section	No exceptions
Without CPD	Oxytocin	Rest for exhaustion

Source: Reprinted from *Labor: Clinical Evaluation and Management*, 2nd ed., by Emanuel A. Friedman, with permission of Appleton-Century-Crofts, © 1978.

Friedman's estimate that CPD accounts for 45 percent of arrested labors (see Table 11-2) is too high. Therefore, experienced midwives are more likely to use expectancy and support (doing nothing medically), therapeutic rest (stopping labor), and (more rarely) conservative means of stimulating labor than Figure 11-1 indicates.

Watch and Wait. Refraining from medical intervention is not the same as "doing nothing." Even if the attendant has good reason not to attempt to change the course of the labor, scrupulous monitoring of the condition of the baby and the mother is essential. Frequent auscultation of the fetal heart should be especially thorough during both contractions and rest periods. The attendant should listen for variability, baseline in the normal range, any abnormal patterns, and the response to fetal movement. The mother's temperature, pulse, and blood pressure should also be carefully monitored. The mother should be well hydrated and without significant ketonuria. If her membranes are ruptured, extra precautions to monitor and prevent infections should be carried out.

Stop the Contractions. Stopping the labor allows the mother, her uterus, and the baby to rest. Morphine is often used for this purpose in the hospital, but this drug is inappropriate for home use. In its place, the combination of alcohol and hydroxyzine pamoate (Vistaril®) by mouth has been used in the home to stop premature labor or help a woman settle down in prolonged latent phase, although its reliability is undocumented. A long hot bath and back rub plus a very restful environment should help put the mother to sleep as the contractions tail off. Stopping labor is generally limited to latent phase, although some midwives favor therapeutic rest by nonmedicinal means in active labor as well.

Sometimes the mother has trouble handling the contractions when she first lies down. When she finally begins to relax, the contractions start to go away. Before the mother tries to sleep she should be very well hydrated, because she will not be drinking while she is asleep. Someone should observe her to confirm that she is sleeping and having only a little or no labor. If she stoically lies in bed trying to sleep but is really having contractions all night long, she will not be having adequate monitoring. Once the woman has been diagnosed to be in active labor an attendant should be in the home (sleeping herself if necessary) even if the labor has been stopped.

Stimulate the Contractions. Stimulating labor, which is less frequently attempted in the home than stopping labor, requires close supervision of the baby's response and the effect on the uterus, as well as very intense labor support for the mother. Therefore the attendant should be present at all times. If the uterus begins to work harder, it will need good hydration and calories. Concerted walking, artificial rupture of membranes (if appropriate dilatation and station, e.g., 6 to 8 cm at +1, are reached), and an enema or castor oil (if the mother's and the baby's conditions seem to allow enough time for it to take effect) are relatively safe techniques of stimulation, although Friedman[39] regards artificial rupture of membranes as contraindicated for this purpose. None of these techniques works consistently; which one will work for a particular woman may be a matter of intuition or trial and error. Nipple stimulation and kissing[40] are also effective, as is strong internal pressure over the rectum. Efforts to correct a malpresentation may be undertaken in conjunction with stimulating labor. To assist a posterior presentation to rotate to anterior, some clinicians suggest that the mother lie on the same side as the fetal back.[41] Others suggest that she lie on the same side as the fetal small parts.[42] The knee-chest or hands-and-knees position may be helpful in pulling the presenting part out of the pelvis to help it rotate.[43] This position should be assumed for at least five consecutive good contractions. The pelvis can be widened by the mother's assuming a deep squat.

Transfer to Hospital. The attendant should take time to prepare the parents concerning the need for transfer and encourage them to feel hopeful that a good birth experience is still possible in the hospital. Before leaving the home, the couple should be given a few moments alone to vent their feelings. The attendant should either drive them or follow them to the hospital in the unlikely event that labor accelerates and delivery occurs en route.

Fetal Distress

The mother in labor at home is frequently in positions that make listening to the baby difficult. She will have to lie down briefly while the fetal heart tones are heard, or else the attendant will have to use an ultrasound monitor. The attendant should be knowledgeable about the controversies surrounding ultrasound[44] and use it only when a regular fetoscope is insufficient (see also Chapter 7). The normal fetal heart rate is between 120 and 160 beats per minute. The following is a brief review of abnormal fetal heart rates and patterns.[45]

- *moderate tachycardia:* baseline of 161 to 180 beats per minute; two recordings 15 minutes apart should prompt consultation and probable transfer.
- *marked tachycardia:* 180 beats per minute and over (could be indicative of infection or mild hypoxia); two recordings 15 minutes apart should prompt consultation and probable transfer.
- *moderate bradycardia:* 100 to 119 beats per minute (common in late second stage); calls for consultation and possible transfer if in first stage.
- *marked bradycardia:* under 100 beats per minute (common in late second stage); calls for consultation and probable transfer if in first stage.
- *minimal variability:* (could mean early fetal distress); two recordings 15 minutes apart should prompt consultation and probable transfer.
- *early deceleration:* Fetal heart rate mirrors the shape of the contraction inversely; deceleration is greatest as contraction peaks; thought to be due to head compression and considered benign. (Deceleration to 80 to 90 beats per minute should be clearly differentiated from the maternal pulse.)
- *late deceleration:* Fetal heart tones slow down late in the contraction, after the peak, with bradycardia persisting beyond the contraction into the rest period; may occur in conjunction with reactive tachycardia and is attributable to uteroplacental insufficiency. The mother is turned on her side and given oxygen at six liters per minute. If not corrected or if another risk factor is already present, transfer is required.

- *variable deceleration:* Heart rate is not reflective of the shape of a contraction and does not keep a consistent pattern from one contraction to the next; may occur randomly between contractions. The baseline may be bradycardia or in the low normal range. A vaginal examination is done immediately. If a prolapsed cord is felt, the fetal head is elevated to remove the pressure. Oxygen (six liters per minute) is given to the mother. She is turned into the knee-chest position, with the attendant keeping a hand on the baby's head. Transfer by ambulance is done immediately. (See discussion of cord prolapse under Problems in Latent Phase.) If the prolapse occurs in second stage and the baby might be deliverable within a few contractions, a large episiotomy is cut and the mother is helped to squat the baby out with all her strength. One must be prepared to resuscitate the baby.

    If a prolapsed cord is not felt, the possibility of an occult prolapse must still be considered. The woman is turned into the knee-chest position and given oxygen as above, and transfer to hospital is initiated.

Other more subtle fetal heart rate patterns (e.g., sinusoidal) are not as diagnostically helpful. (See Kruse[46] for a more detailed discussion of fetal heart rate patterns.)

Meconium Staining

Both the interpretation and the management of meconium staining are controversial. Some newborns have bowel movements once in four days, others 20 times in one day. Since the anal sphincter is anatomically the same before birth as after, it follows that some infants must be predisposed to pass the contents of their bowels much more readily, given similar stimulation, than others. Some fetuses, therefore, may pass meconium at the slightest insult, while others may need to be severely compromised before their anal sphincters react. A study correlating the passage of meconium in labor with the bowel habits of newborns would be useful.

Clearly, meconium should be considered a sign of *possible* distress and used with other parameters in determining the management of a given labor and the question of transfer. The thicker its texture and the earlier it appears, the more likely it is that meconium signifies fetal distress.[47] In any event, meconium does present a danger to the newborn because of possible aspiration. A healthy baby without hypoxia can be damaged by sequelae of meconium aspiration, such as chemical pneumonia. A hypoxic baby who aspirates may suffer even more serious complications (e.g., respiratory distress, persistent fetal circulation).

If meconium is present, the attendant should have the DeLee suction trap ready at delivery. (Some models such as the Bard-Parker infant suction set must have the cap screwed tightly onto the trap.) Between the birth of the head and that of the shoulders, the mother must refrain from pushing while the attendant thoroughly but gently suctions the baby's oropharynx. If a considerable amount of meconium is found, direct visualization of and suctioning below the vocal cords is advisable (see Chapter 12).

If the baby has any respiratory difficulties related to meconium, or if meconium is found below the cords, the baby should be transferred to a neonatal intensive-care unit.

Shoulder Dystocia

The term *shoulder dystocia* is used to describe a delay or difficulty in delivering the baby's shoulders. It is seen more commonly with protracted active phase dilatation and prolonged descent patterns. Other findings are retraction of the head (which probably is large) against the perineum and lack of (or slow) restitution. When shoulder dystocia is diagnosed, the following steps are taken:

1. If the first contraction after the head is born does not quickly result in spontaneous delivery of the shoulders, gentle pressure is applied on the baby's head toward the mother's rectum with the contraction to bring the anterior shoulder under the symphysis.
2. If the shoulders are still not born when the first contraction ends, one of the following maneuvers is tried:
   a. Before the next contraction, the mother's legs are hyperflexed up against her chest and an attempt is made to rotate the anterior shoulder into the oblique angle. Suprapubic pressure is helpful. Some authorities believe that fundal pressure (in conjunction with suprapubic) adds to the rotational and expulsive forces.[48] During the contraction the mother is assisted to push very hard and the downward traction on the baby's head is repeated.
   b. The mother is rotated either to her hands and knees[49] or to a full squatting position, which often brings the baby's shoulders out without further manipulation.
3. If the shoulders are still undelivered after the second contraction, a large mediolateral (sometimes bilateral) episiotomy is cut and then the corkscrew maneuver[50] is performed and downward traction is repeated.

4. If unsuccessful, the attendant should try to deliver the posterior shoulder by reaching into the vagina and sweeping the posterior arm across the baby's chest and out of the vagina. Then an attempt to either deliver the anterior arm or rotate the baby 180 degrees and deliver the other shoulder the same way is made.
5. If unsuccessful, the attendant should break the baby's clavicle.

Face Presentation

A face presentation is recognized by palpating the orbits of the skull, the mouth, and the back of the fontanels.[51,52]

1. If the presentation is mentum posterior, transfer to the hospital is required.
2. If the presentation is anterior, a transfer is made if there is time. If a decision is made to attempt delivery at home (which is rarely wise), monitoring for fetal distress is intensified. When the face is being born, extension is maintained until the chin is born under the symphysis.[53] The rest of the face is then born by flexion. If the baby's face is moulded, one must reassure parents that it will return to normal contours.

Breech Delivery

1. Prenatal screening should detect almost all breeches (see Chapter 7).[54,55] An abdominal examination should be done routinely in early labor to rule out the rest. If the presentation is discovered in early labor, an unhurried transfer to the hospital can take place.
2. If delivery in the home is unpreventable because of improper screening or distance from the hospital, resuscitation is prepared for, the receiving blankets are warmed, and an ambulance is called to stand by. (Theoretically, the situation should never be allowed to reach this point, but if the baby's legs come out first, it is better to deliver at home than to risk a difficult delivery in an ambulance.)
3. The mother is assisted to urinate in a towel or over a pot.
4. The attendant should make sure that the cervix is *completely* dilated before permitting the mother to push. It is important to check that there is no prolapsed cord.
5. Either the supported squat of Odent[56] (described earlier in this chapter), which allows the maximum chance of a totally spontaneous delivery, or the Lamaze or dorsal position (with two people

holding the mother's legs wide apart), which allows the attendant the most room to maneuver is used.
6. An episiotomy is performed unless the perineum is relaxed and the baby is not too large.
7. The baby's body is kept warm as it is born.
8. When the legs and trunk up to the umbilicus are born, a loop of cord is pulled down to give it slack so that it will not be pulled too tight during other maneuvers.
9. The baby's body is rotated gently from side to side to assist the birth of the shoulders. The baby's back should be kept facing anterior.
10. The baby's body is allowed to hang down. Someone else should give suprapubic pressure to assist in flexing the head when the nape of the neck (hairline) appears.
11. The baby's body is lifted upward to follow the curve of Carus as the lower face sweeps the perineum.
12. An airway is cleared as soon as possible.
13. The rest of the head is delivered slowly and gently if breathing is established.
14. Preparations are made to give oxygen and/or assisted ventilation if necessary.
15. The baby is evaluated as soon as possible (see Chapter 12).

Multiple Delivery

1. Every effort should be made to diagnose twins (or other multiples) prenatally.[57]
2. If multiple birth is discovered in labor, transfer to a hospital is required.
3. If twins are discovered only when delivery is imminent, the birth of the first child should proceed normally if the head is down. An ambulance should be called to stand by. If the first baby is not a vertex presentation, the presenting part is held off the pelvic floor manually to delay the delivery and transfer is made by ambulance.
4. After the birth of the first twin, the cord is immediately clamped and cut.
5. If the second twin is not discovered until after the first twin is delivered, the cord of the first twin is clamped as soon as twins are suspected. The second fetal heart is monitored frequently. The presentation and position of the second twin are ascertained. If the presentation is not a vertex, transfer is required immediately unless

one is very experienced with breech deliveries or internal version of transverse lie.

6. An intravenous line is started if birth in the home is likely.
7. A wait of up to 15 minutes is allowed for the presentation of the second twin. The presenting part is guided into the pelvis with fundal pressure and manipulation of the presenting part internally with a hand inserted in the vagina. The second set of membranes is ruptured, and a check is made to ascertain that no cord prolapses.
8. The mother is told to push.
9. If contractions do not resume, nipple stimulation (by the first twin or the father) and rectal pressure are tried.
10. When the second twin delivers, its cord is clamped with two hemostats for identification.
11. If the second twin is not delivered in 30 minutes or if the cervix starts to close up again, transport in an ambulance is made. Preparations are made for possible delivery in the ambulance. The first twin must not be forgotten.
12. Steps 4 through 11 are repeated for as many babies as necessary.
13. Postpartum hemorrhage is possible. "Active management" of the third stage (10 IU oxytocin (Pitocin®) with anterior shoulder of last baby and Brandt-Andrews technique of assisted delivery of placenta[58]) should be considered. Manual removal of the placentas may be necessary.
14. If all babies and mother are well, placentas delivered intact, and the fundus firm, the ambulance can be dismissed. If there is any question at all about the situation, transfer is advised.
15. Both (or all) babies are carefully evaluated. The placentas and membranes are examined to determine whether the twins are monozygotic or dizygotic.
16. To help prevent hemorrhage, the mother is encouraged to have the twins nurse continually, or for as long as they will.
17. The mother is given ergonovine maleate (Ergotrate Maleate®) tablets, 0.2 mg, to take orally every 6 hours for 24 hours (even in the absence of the bleeding that is the usual indication for Ergotrate).

Third-Stage Complications

It is essential that a home birth service have a well elaborated protocol for management of the third stage, one that allows for the various contingencies that may occur, since it is in this stage that serious complications leading to maternal morbidity and mortality are most likely to occur.[59,60] The following is the protocol used in the authors' practice:

Hemorrhage Before Placenta Is Delivered

1. Diagnosis includes bleeding in excess of the usual separation bleeding, either a larger amount or a steady trickle. Technically, a hemorrhage is defined as bleeding over 500 ml, but vigilance should begin earlier in the home.
2. Whether the placenta has separated is ascertained.
3. If separation clearly has occurred, the placenta is delivered immediately with Brandt-Andrews maneuver.
4. If the placenta has not clearly separated but the bleeding continues, the uterus is massaged to stimulate a strong contraction and the Brandt-Andrews maneuver is tried.
5. If the placenta still does not deliver and the bleeding persists, 10 IU oxytocin (Pitocin®) is given intramuscularly and transfer is immediate. If there is shock or if time considerations (rate of bleeding versus distance to hospital) make transfer inadvisable, intravenous therapy is begun and manual removal is performed. As soon as the placenta is delivered, 10 IU oxytocin should be added to the intravenous line. If manual removal must be performed in the home without an intravenous line, the oxytocin may be given intramuscularly first because the added time taken for absorption by that route allows time for the procedure. Emergency manual removal in the home does not eliminate the need for transfer due to excessive blood loss.
6. Bimanual compression can be used to control bleeding in transit. The mother is given oxygen and monitored carefully.
7. If the placenta delivers but is not intact, and if bleeding has not stopped, the uterus is explored. If this skill is not known, oxytocin is given and transfer is immediate. If bleeding has stopped, transfer is made to hospital for uterine exploration, but oxytocin is not given.
8. Once the placenta delivers, blood loss is evaluated according to the criteria in the following section.

Hemorrhage After Placenta Is Delivered

1. The most likely cause of hemorrhage is uterine atony. The uterus should be massaged until it contracts well.
2. If the uterus does not contract, bimanual compression is done and oxytocin is given intramuscularly. An assistant monitors the mother's pulse and blood pressure.
3. If the uterus contracts but does not stay well contracted, with resultant continuation of bleeding, the attendant should try to express clots from the uterus abdominally or vaginally and then give methylergonovine (Methergine®), 0.2 mg, intramuscularly.

4. If the uterus still does not contract or hold well, an ambulance is called and the mother is transferred. Bimanual compression is performed en route to the hospital.
5. If the uterus contracts and holds well but bleeding continues, the woman is examined for cervical or vaginal tears. Bleeders are clamped with small hemostats and transfer to hospital is made if the repair cannot be accomplished at home.[61]
6. Estimated blood loss is assessed as follows:
   a. Blood loss of 500 ml or less with good clinical condition requires no additional measures.
   b. Blood loss of 500 to 1,000 ml with stable clinical condition after diagnosis and treatment requires a four-hour period of observation at home.
   c. Blood loss of more than 1,000 ml is an indication for intravenous therapy and hospitalization for consideration of blood transfusion. If the woman's condition is clinically unstable or undiagnosed, transfer to the hospital with an intravenous line in place is indicated. Emergency transport service and hospital care backup should be notified at the outset of the initial home management.
7. If the mother is not transferred to the hospital, she may be given ergonovine maleate (Ergotrate Maleate®) tablets, 0.2 mg, to take orally every 6 hours for 24 hours (or as needed) for follow-up of hemorrhage or heavy bleeding.

Retained Placenta Without Bleeding

1. A time limit of 45 minutes for the third stage can be considered safe if access to hospitals is good. Some practitioners are willing to wait longer, provided that no overt bleeding occurs and there are no signs of concealed bleeding.
2. A vaginal examination may reveal the placenta to be sitting in the lower segment, the cervix, or the vagina. The attendant may be able to grasp the placenta manually in the upper vagina. In these cases, the Brandt-Andrews maneuver can be tried with a well-contracted uterus.
3. If these measures fail, transfer is indicated. Manual removal of the placenta in the home, without the added incentive of hemorrhage, is too risky. In addition to the other risks of manual removal (e.g., infection, uterine perforation, technical difficulties in accomplishing complete removal, difficulties presented by lack of anesthesia), the possibility of placenta accreta can bring about sudden, uncontrollable bleeding.

Uterine Inversion

Uterine inversion is an extremely rare obstetric disaster. The attendant should consult standard textbooks so as to become familiar with the emergency treatment of this complication but even more familiar with its prevention.[62,63]

*Obstacles to Appropriate Decision Making in Third-Stage
Complications*

However precise the protocols and however technically well-prepared the attendant, good clinical judgment can be undermined by commonly experienced emotional reactions such as the following:

The New Parents' Reaction. The overwhelming emotional and physical relief at the birth of the baby frequently leaves the new parents unprepared to accept that there is still more work to do. When a large amount of bleeding fails to show itself dramatically, the attendant's announcement of a hemorrhage may seem unbelievable, especially if the mother still feels well. Conversely, when a small amount of bleeding does show itself dramatically, the family (and particularly the new father) may be alarmed out of proportion to the severity of the bleeding.

The Attendant's Reaction. The effect on the attendant may be equally dramatic.

- *fear:* The prospect of a maternal death is so frightening and culturally unacceptable that even an experienced attendant may begin to sweat, shake, and otherwise manifest fear. Attendants should remind themselves that the physical signs of fear show the body's response of mobilizing its resources in the face of danger.
- *fatigue:* A complication in third stage may find the attendant already drained after a long labor. The importance of teamwork between attendants is evident here.

Reluctance to Leave the Home. If the birth has been satisfying, if everyone is tired, if the hemorrhage seems to be under control, if the response from the hospital may be equivocal if a transfer is made—these are all factors that weigh against transfer in the minds and emotions of both the family and the attendant. In some instances these factors may serve to prevent an unnecessary transfer. In other instances they may prevent a timely transfer and bring about a later, more emergent, more risky, and more stressful transfer.

The only way to remove these obstacles is to discuss them openly. The attendants should verbalize their concerns and reactions, acknowledging fear and other emotions, as well as discussing the technical merits of different options.

Shock

There are many possible causes of shock in a home birth. The different types of shock (e.g., endotoxic, cardiogenic, hemorrhagic, anaphylactic) should be familiar to the attendant.

The signs and symptoms of shock from whatever cause include extreme hypotension, tachycardia, an orthostatic pulse[64] (a rise of 10 beats per minute or a drop in systolic blood pressure of 10 mm Hg from the supine to the sitting position), tachypnea, cold clammy skin, a feeling of weakness, dizziness, nausea, and ringing in the ears.

Treatment for shock is as follows:

1. An ambulance is called immediately and the ambulance attendants are notified that the woman appears to be in shock.
2. An assistant monitors the woman's pulse and blood pressure every 5 to 10 minutes.
3. It is important to keep talking to the woman and see that she responds and is reassured.
4. An intravenous line with parenteral fluids such as lactated Ringer's is started using a large bore needle or intravenous catheter (e.g., 16 to 18 gauge).
5. The mother's legs are elevated and her head is lowered.
6. The woman is covered with blankets and given six liters per minute of oxygen by nasal cannula or mask. If hemorrhage has been profuse, the attendant should piggyback the intravenous line with serum albumin or other plasma expanders. If hemorrhage continues, aortic compression is performed en route to the hospital. In this procedure the abdominal aorta is compressed against the spine by an assistant's fist pressed inward just above the umbilicus. Aortic compression may reduce the amount of blood lost during uncontrollable hemorrhage while awaiting an ambulance and during transport.[65] Bimanual compression is continued if possible.
7. If the woman becomes unconscious, an airway is inserted and cardiopulmonary resuscitation is given as needed.

USEFUL CLINICAL SKILLS

Castor Oil Induction

Castor oil induction has been found to be useful in clinical experience, although its effectiveness has not been documented in controlled trials.

1. Two tablespoons of unflavored castor oil are given in six to eight ounces of juice blended with 1 ounce of hard liquor (to promote tension release and relaxation before the castor oil takes effect). The mother should take a long, hot, steaming bath and try to rest.
2. One hour later, two more tablespoons of castor oil in juice and an enema are given. Since stimulation is now beginning in earnest, hard liquor is no longer used. The mother should walk around as much as possible.
3. One hour later, administration of the castor oil in juice is repeated. Diarrhea will begin soon, and contractions should commence in four to six hours.

Suturing

1. The mother is placed in approximated lithotomy position on the edge of her bed with her feet on chairs or stools. An armchair with armrests that will support her legs is an alternative.
2. The attendant should make an effort to get comfortable and to obtain good lighting. These factors will affect how well the repair turns out. An assistant may need to put on a sterile glove to hold the mother's labia apart, while holding a flashlight in the other hand to provide extra lighting.
3. A decision is made as to what suturing needs to be done and whether any attendant present is competent to do it. The woman deserves to have her pelvic floor returned to its proper anatomy and, if necessary, will find a brief trip to the hospital well worth her while.
4. The floor is protected with disposable underpads and a place for a sterile field that will not be disturbed is found. Ample supplies of suture material should be on hand.
5. The vulva and perineum are cleansed as thoroughly as possible with antiseptic solution. Too much draping is probably counterproductive at home, without stirrups and a delivery table.
6. The repair is begun. Home birth attendants may find hand ties more convenient than instrument ties because there may be less room to maneuver at home.
7. It is especially important to be attentive to possible reactions to local anesthesia. These are usually handled by oxygen administration, atropine for prolonged bradycardia (vasovagal reactions), leg elevation, intravenous fluids for volume expansion, anticonvulsants (if available) for seizures, epinephrine for anaphylactic reactions, and intubation for apnea or respiratory failure. Mild transitory reactions may require nothing more than reassurance and judicious monitoring

of pulse, blood pressure, respirations, and level of consciousness. In more severe cases an ambulance should be called in case transport to hospital is required.

Intravenous Therapy in the Home

A birth in which intravenous therapy is required should not be completed in the home. Some home birth attendants do not even carry intravenous fluids and equipment; instead, they arrange for infusion to begin in the ambulance on the way to the hospital. Ideally, the attendant should be prepared to start an intravenous line in the home. However, if intravenous therapy is required, preparations for transfer should be underway. Intravenous therapy may be used in the home to help stabilize a woman's condition for safe transfer. Only very rarely does it result in reassessment of the decision to transfer.

TRANSFER TO THE HOSPITAL

The successful management of transfers from home to hospital during labor depends on careful preparation before labor begins. As discussed in Chapter 7, prenatal care for home births includes informing the family of the criteria for transfer and reaching clear agreement about how the decision will be made and what prerogatives the attendants reserve for themselves. The attendants should identify the hospital where they are most comfortable, clinically and philosophically, and where the staff (including obstetricians, anesthesiologists, neonatologists, and nurses) is most flexible in dealing with issues of concern to families and practitioners involved in home birth. Backup relationships with this hospital should be established as outlined in Chapter 6. This will be the hospital of choice for nonemergency transfers. For emergency transfers (which occur very infrequently), the closest hospital is used.

If transfer occurs after delivery of the baby and/or placenta, they should accompany the mother to the hospital.

Transfer by Ambulance

1. Ambulance transport from the home should be prearranged and the telephone number of the ambulance service posted near every telephone. The address of the home and the telephone numbers of physicians and hospitals for backup should be posted as well.

2. How quickly transfer may need to be accomplished is determined. If a potentially serious problem might occur, such as uterine rupture, the ambulance should be called well before it is actually needed. If it is a false alarm, the ambulance can be dismissed.
3. An assistant calls the ambulance. It is important to be succinct and to indicate briefly what is happening, what is needed, where the woman is to be transferred, and who the physician in charge will be. Some companies ask for the caller's telephone number and then call back to verify the caller's seriousness.
4. The hospital and the backup physician are called.
5. The mother and/or the baby are stabilized for transport. The steps being taken are explained at all times.
6. The attendant accompanies the parents in the ambulance if possible and continues to provide medical assistance unless the ambulance attendant is better qualified to do so. If the ambulance attendant provides inappropriate treatment, a calm but firm display of skill, knowledge, and credentials usually establishes control.

Transfer by Car

1. If the transfer is not a hurried one, there will be time for preparation for a hospital birth. The parents are reminded to bring a safety seat for bringing the baby home. They should be allowed time to say goodbye to friends or family who are not coming. Often those friends who have attended the labor will come along, if only to wait in the lobby and see the baby through the nursery window.
2. The attendant should follow the parents' car to the hospital. The mother will also need labor support in the car if she is still having contractions. The parents should be instructed to pull over if there are any problems so that the attendant with the kit will be right there.

In the Hospital

The attendant should make introductions in the hospital and assist with the care and the labor support (see Chapter 6). If the mother must stay in the hospital, she will want her baby admitted. If she will only be there briefly, the hospital may allow the baby to come in as a "visitor." This may have to be negotiated at the time of admission.

INFORMED CONSENT AND HOME BIRTH

In the home as well as the hospital, prospective parents have a right to all relevant information about the mother's and the baby's conditions and the care given them. They have a right to know what alternative treatments are available for a given condition (including what the traditional medical treatment is if the attendant is suggesting a nontraditional treatment). In a home birth much of the informed consent process takes place in the prenatal briefings (described in Chapter 7) on the risks and benefits of home birth itself as well as on those of specific procedures that differ from standard obstetric practice. Nonetheless, the informed consent requirements should be kept in mind when situations requiring clinical choices arise during labor. The woman and her partner do not need to know every anxious thought that crosses the attendant's mind, but they must be informed if there is any real possibility of a problem. The attendant will find his or her own way to present this necessary information without destroying the mother's confidence in her ability to give birth normally.

As indicated in Chapter 4, a birth attendant may refuse to go to the home of a family that has rejected the attendant's recommendation of hospital care. The hospital and the backup physician should be informed of this situation immediately. Once in the home, however, the birth attendant must not leave even if the family refuses treatment or transfer. To do so is called *abandonment,* which is a serious ethical and legal issue. The attendant should alert the hospital and the backup physician immediately of this turn of events. The parents should be fully informed of the consequences of their actions, but all possible assistance (that they will accept) should be given them.

NOTES

1. Harold Bursztajn et al., *Medical Choices, Medical Chances: How Patients, Families, and Physicians Can Cope With Uncertainty* (New York: Delacorte Press/Seymour Lawrence, 1981), pp. 20–84, 349–388.

2. Gayle Peterson, *Birthing Normally: A Personal Growth Approach to Childbirth* (Berkeley, Calif.: Mindbody Press, 1981), pp.63–67.

3. Margaret F. Myles, *Textbook for Midwives*, 8th ed. (Edinburgh: Churchill Livingstone, 1975), pp. 111–113.

4. Denis Cavanagh, Ralph E. Woods, and Timothy C.F. O'Connor, *Obstetric Emergencies,* 2nd ed. (Hagerstown, Md.: Harper & Row, 1978), p. 79.

5. James A. O'Leary, Hiram W. Mendenhall, and George C. Andrinopoulos, "Comparison of Auditory Versus Electronic Assessment of Antenatal Fetal Welfare," *Obstetrics and Gynecology* 56 (1980): 244–246.

6. Gregory C. Starks, "Correlation of Meconium-Stained Amniotic Fluid, Early Intrapartum Fetal pHs and Apgar Scores as Predictors of Perinatal Outcome," *Obstetrics and Gynecology* 56 (1980): 604–609.

7. Albert D. Haverkamp et al., "The Evaluation of Continuous Fetal Heart Rate Monitoring in High-Risk Pregnancy," *American Journal of Obstetrics and Gynecology* 125 (1976): 310–320.

8. William A. Check,"Electronic Fetal Monitoring: How Necessary?" *Journal of the American Medical Association* 241 (1979): 1772–1774.

9. Helen Varney, *Nurse-Midwifery* (Boston: Blackwell Scientific Publications, 1980), pp. 178–179.

10. William S. Freeman, "Pre-eclampsia: What to Do and When,"*PriCare* 11 (1979): 637–642.

11. Varney, *Nurse-Midwifery*, p. 521.

12. Jenifer M. Fleming, "Children at Birth: A Guide to Preparing Children for the Birth of a Sibling at Home or in a Birthing Room" (Cambridge, Mass.: Birth Day, 1980).

13. Cavanagh, Woods, and O'Connor, *Obstetric Emergencies*, p. 348.

14. Laurel Robertson, Carol Flinders, and Bronwen Godfrey, *Laurel's Kitchen* (New York: Bantam, 1978), p. 586.

15. Ibid., p. 568.

16. John A. Read et al., "Urinary Bladder Distention: Effect on Labor and Uterine Activity," *Obstetrics and Gynecology* 56 (1980): 565–570.

17. Isaac N. Mitre, "The Influence of Maternal Position on Duration of the Active Phase of Labor," *International Journal of Gynecology and Obstetrics* 12 (1974): 181–183.

18. Carlos Mendez-Bauer et al.,"Effects of Standing Position on Spontaneous Uterine Contractility and Other Aspects of Labor," *Journal of Perinatal Medicine* 3 (1975): 89–100.

19. Peter M. Dunn, "Obstetric Delivery Today: For Better or For Worse?" *Lancet* 1 (1976): 790–793.

20. A.M. Flynn et al., "Ambulation in Labour," *British Medical Journal* 2 (1978): 591–593.

21. Roberto Caldeyro-Barcia, "The Influence of Maternal Position on Time of Spontaneous Rupture of the Membranes, Progress of Labor, and Fetal Head Compression," *Birth and the Family Journal* 6 (1979): 7–15.

22. John A. Read, Frank C. Miller, and Richard H. Paul, "Randomized Trial of Ambulation vs. Oxytocin for Labor Enhancement: A Preliminary Report," *American Journal of Obstetrics and Gynecology* 139 (1981): 669–672.

23. Varney, *Nurse-Midwifery*, p. 204.

24. Elizabeth Davis, *A Guide to Midwifery: Hearts and Hands* (Santa Fe: John Muir Publications, 1981), pp. 107–108.

25. Elizabeth Noble,"Controversies in Maternal Effort During Labor and Delivery," *Journal of Nurse-Midwifery* 26, no. 2 (March/April 1981): 13–22.

26. Roberto Caldeyro-Barcia, "Physiological and Psychological Bases for the Modern and Humanized Management of Normal Labor." Paper presented at the International Year of the Child Commemorative Congress, Tokyo, Japan, October 21–22, 1979.

27. Katherine Camacho Carr, "Obstetrical Practices Which Protect Against Neonatal Morbidity: Focus on Maternal Position in Labor and Birth," *Birth and the Family Journal* 7 (1980): 249–254.

28. Michel Odent, "The Evolution of Obstetrics at Pithiviers," *Birth and the Family Journal* 8 (1981): 7–15.

29. Ibid.

30. Varney, *Nurse-Midwifery*, p. 213.

31. Mary Lee Ingbar et al., "Choosing Services for Maternity Care and Childbirth: A Case Study" (Worcester, Mass.: University of Massachusetts Medical School, Department of Family and Community Medicine, 1980), pp. III, 4–11.

32. Peterson, *Birthing Normally*, pp. 115–130.

33. Emanuel A. Friedman, *Labor: Clinical Evaluation and Management*, 2nd ed. (New York: Appleton-Century-Crofts, 1978), p. 33.

34. Ibid., pp. 63, 67–69.

35. Ibid.

36. Ibid.

37. Harry Oxorn and William R. Foote, *Human Labor and Birth*, 3rd ed. (New York: Appleton-Century-Crofts, 1975), pp.468–484.

38. Naseem Jagani et al., "The Predictability of Labor Outcome From a Comparison of Birth Weight and X-ray Pelvimetry," *American Journal of Obstetrics and Gynecology* 139 (1981): 507–511.

39. Friedman, *Labor*, pp. 341–342.

40. Ina May Gaskin, *Spiritual Midwifery* (Summertown, Tenn.: The Book Publishing Co., 1978), pp. 349, 443.

41. Varney, *Nurse-Midwifery*, p. 186.

42. Oxorn and Foote, *Human Labor and Birth*, p. 144.

43. Davis, *Guide to Midwifery*, p. 97.

44. Lewis H. Nelson and Frederick Kremkau, "Real-time Diagnostic Ultrasound in Obstetrics," *American Family Physician* 25, no. 1 (January 1982): 149–156.

45. Varney, *Nurse-Midwifery*, pp. 239–243.

46. Jerry Kruse, "Electronic Fetal Monitoring During Labor," *Journal of Family Practice* 15 (1982): 35–42.

47. Starks,"Correlation of Meconium-Stained Amniotic Fluid," pp. 604–609.

48. Herbert G. Hopwood, Jr., "Shoulder Dystocia: Fifteen Years' Experience in a Community Hospital," *American Journal of Obstetrics and Gynecology* 144 (1982): 162–166.

49. Gaskin, *Spiritual Midwifery*, p. 364.

50. Oxorn and Foote, *Human Labor and Birth*, pp. 254–255.

51. Thomas J. Benedetti, Richard I. Lowensohn, and Al M. Truscott,"Face Presentation at Term," *Obstetrics and Gynecology* 55 (1980): 199–202.

52. Patrick Duff, "Diagnosis and Management of Face Presentation," *Obstetrics and Gynecology* 57 (1981): 105–112.

53. Varney, *Nurse-Midwifery*, pp. 253–255.

54. Ibid., pp. 255–261.

55. Oxorn and Foote, *Human Labor and Birth*, pp. 193–224.

56. Odent, "The Evolution of Obstetrics," pp. 7–15.

57. Varney, *Nurse-Midwifery*, pp. 262–263.

58. Ibid., pp. 268–269.

59. Ibid., pp. 273–275.

60. Cavanagh, Woods, and O'Connor, *Obstetric Emergencies*, pp. 293–301.

61. Jack A. Pritchard and Paul C. MacDonald, *Williams' Obstetrics*, 15th ed. (New York: Appleton-Century-Crofts, 1976), pp. 727–730.

62. Varney, *Nurse-Midwifery*, pp. 274–275.

63. Oxorn and Foote, *Human Labor and Birth*, pp. 435–438.

64. Pritchard and MacDonald, *Williams' Obstetrics*, p. 402.

65. Oxorn and Foote, *Human Labor and Birth*, p. 402.

Chapter 12

Immediate Care of the Newborn

Principal Author: Richard I. Feinbloom, M.D.

In the great majority of births at home, the infant is in excellent condition and the mood is one of celebration. In recent years the phenomenon of early infant-parent bonding has been given much attention. There has been a reaffirmation of the traditional wisdom that it is desirable for babies and their parents to have early uninhibited contact.[1] In fact, interference with such contact in hospitals was an important impetus to the home birth movement. In a home birth the parents should be viewed as being in charge during the postpartum period; the attendants are present to advise, to assist, and to intervene only if necessary.

However, the potential always exists for life-threatening cardiorespiratory depression, which requires immediate intervention. The first part of this chapter focuses on this problem. The challenge for the attendant is to be familiar with the techniques of resuscitation and to maintain the requisite skills even though their exercise is infrequently required. The account that follows assumes that two attendants are present and would need to be modified if only one were involved.

PREPARATORY MEASURES

The room temperature should be at least 70 degrees. A heating pad can be warmed in readiness for the birth. Blankets, Kelly clamps, scissors, bulb syringe, and cord tie should be readily at hand. The instruments should be sterilized; this can be done in a pot supplied by the family. The covered pot is kept in the room used for the birth.

The oxygen tank valve is opened so that turning the control dial alone is enough to initiate flow. Items regularly used for newborn care are removed from the birth kit and placed in or near the birthing room (see complete inventory in Chapter 10).

There are several kinds of ventilating bags available. Attendants are advised to check with anesthesiologists in their areas. The authors have had good results with the Penlon-Cardiff infant inflating bag. This bag is designed to minimize the possibility of excessive pressure and lung rupture whether the lungs are collapsed or expanded.

GRADED CARE OF THE NEWBORN ACCORDING TO APGAR SCORE

The Apgar score is a tested way to classify infants according to the level of immediate care required.[2] It is determined at 1 and 5 minutes after birth. The score is not intended to lead to reflex responses by the attendants. Rather, the attendants should gauge the direction in which the score is moving. For example, if depressed respiration seems to be improving spontaneously, resuscitation efforts need not be instituted simply because the score was initially depressed.

The Apgar score consists of five measures of newborn functioning and developmental status on which (as shown in Table 12-1) the infant is given a rating from 0 to 2. Thus, the overall Apgar score may range from 0 to 10. Full-term babies born without anesthesia and without evident complications almost always have a high Apgar score. The protocol given in Exhibit 12-1 indicates appropriate clinical responses for a given range of

Table 12-1 The Apgar Score

Sign	Score		
	0	1	2
Heart rate	Absent	Under 100 beats per minute	Over 100 beats per minute
Respiratory effort	Absent	Slow (irregular)	Good crying
Muscle tone	Limp	Some flexion of extremities	Active motion
Reflex irritability	No response	Grimace	Cough or sneeze
Color	Blue, pale	Pink body, blue extremities	All pink

Source: Reprinted from "A Proposal for a New Method of Evaluation of the Newborn Infant," by Virginia Apgar, *Anesthesia and Analgesia* vol. 32, pp. 260–267, with permission of the International Anesthesia Research Society, © 1953.

Exhibit 12-1 Appropriate Clinical Responses According to Apgar Score

No Asphyxia (Apgar 8–10)
1. If necessary, suction upper airway with bulb syringe with baby's head held slightly lower than its body; cover with blankets including the head; hand baby to mother (in some births, mother herself will have caught the baby); hold baby at the level of the uterus for 45 seconds or place baby on mother's abdomen to allow achievement of optimal blood volume; do not "strip" the blood from the umbilical cord; cut and tie the cord; put infant to breast (to promote uterine contractions, to provide infant with nourishment, and to foster early bonding); obtain a sample of cord blood for metabolic screening (usually dripped directly onto a card provided by the laboratory). For babies of Rh-negative mothers with Rh-positive fathers, collect a tube of cord blood. Draw a sample of the mother's blood and send both tubes to the laboratory for type and cross-match for RhoGAM as needed.
2. As long as the Apgar score remains 8 and above no further measures need to be taken. At a time convenient to family and attendant (usually within an hour after the birth) the screening physical examination described later in this chapter is performed; eyes are treated (without flushing) with silver nitrate, erythromycin, or tetracycline; and vitamin K is given as needed (see Chapter 7). Problems requiring further care are identified and planned for.

Mild Asphyxia (Apgar 5–7)
1. Stimulation. Gentle slapping of the feet and rubbing of the back is the only stimulation needed.
2. Oxygen. The infant should be provided an oxygen-enriched environment by placing the face mask lightly over the mouth and nose and providing constant oxygen flow. An infant who has not established adequate respiration by five minutes may require bag and mask ventilation.

Moderate Asphyxia (Apgar 3–5)
1. Cut the cord immediately to prevent fetoplacental transfusion. Cutting the cord will also free the baby so that the attendants can move to a nearby hard surface for resuscitative efforts. The prewarmed heating pad should cover the surface used.
2. Suction the oropharynx and nose with the DeLee catheter. If meconium has been passed, also suction the trachea, as described later in this chapter.
3. Begin bag and mask ventilation with 100 percent oxygen. The mask is firmly applied with the thumb and index finger of the left hand, and the bag is compressed with the right hand. The left hand maintains the head in slight extension on the neck. Marked extension will obstruct the airway.
4. After initial chest expansion occurs, quick short bursts of oxygen are administered. The recommended rate is 30 to 40 per minute.[3]

Severe Asphyxia (Apgar 0–2)
Failure of measures described above to increase the heart rate or improve the color necessitates tracheal intubation and the calling in of an ambulance for transfer to hospital.

Asystole or Bradycardia (regardless of Apgar score)
1. Perform external cardiac massage. Face the infant from foot to head, placing both thumbs at the junction of the middle and lower thirds of the sternum with the fingers wrapped around the back of the chest. With the thumbs depressing the sternum approximately two thirds of the distance to the vertebral column, compress and release the sternum 100 times per minute. Observe the results of the massage by palpating the femoral or umbilical cord pulse.

Apgar scores, with the 8 to 10 range applying to the majority of babies born at home.

RESUSCITATION OF THE NEWBORN

In the vast majority of cases, the resuscitation of the severely asphyxiated newborn requires only suction, ventilation, and cardiac massage (the "ABCs" of resuscitation: *a*irway, *b*reathing, and *c*irculation). Nonetheless, it is highly advantageous for home birth attendants to become skilled in intubating newborns. Intubation allows for visualization and removal of meconium below the cords, insertion of an endotracheal tube for administration of oxygen, and stabilization of the newborn for transport to an intensive-care center. When these measures are insufficient, the umbilical vein should be catheterized to facilitate administration of fluid and medications to combat shock and acidosis.

All of the resuscitative procedures discussed here require practice. Screening for home birth is designed to provide the attendant with only very infrequent opportunities to practice these skills in the home. Therefore, unless the home birth attendants also work in hospital settings involving many births, including those of premature babies (the group most needing resuscitative efforts), it is unlikely they will have sufficient exposure to asphyxiated newborns to maintain skills in resuscitation.

Resuscitation drills should be held periodically. Kittens anesthetized with ketamine can be used for practicing intubation.[4] Placentas with attached umbilical cords can be used for practicing umbilical vein catheterization.

It is also important for the attendants to have a definite plan in mind for allocating the tasks involved in resuscitation and to rehearse who does what.

As indicated in the above protocol, infants who are severely asphyxiated should be taken to the hospital even if resuscitative efforts are successful. They are vulnerable to too many serious complications (e.g., infection, development of persistent fetal circulation) to justify remaining at home. In transferring infants with unstable cardiorespiratory function who may need continued care, use of an ambulance service is advised so that resuscitative efforts can proceed without the distractions involved in transportation by private automobile.

Umbilical Vein Catheterization

When the usual resuscitative measures thus far described do not produce the desired results, and when available resources (including trained personnel) and time permit, the umbilical vein is catheterized while mechanical ventilation and cardiac massage are continued. The following solutions are injected in sequence, with the end point that of normal cardiac output as signified by return of the heart rate to 100 beats per minute or above:

1. Sodium bicarbonate—2 mEq/kg (2 ml of a 1 mEq/ml solution) diluted with an equal amount of 10% dextrose in water is administered slowly over 10 minutes (50% dextrose and water can be diluted to 25% by mixing with an equal amount of sterile water; when this 25% solution is diluted one-to-one with an equal quantity of bicarbonate, the resulting dextrose concentration is an acceptable 12.5%).
2. Epinephrine, 1:10,000—0.5 to 1.0 ml is given quickly for asystole or bradycardia.
3. Calcium gluconate, 10%—2 ml is given *slowly* over several minutes.

Shock

Shock in the infant results from significant intrapartum blood loss due to placental separation with fetoplacental or fetomaternal hemorrhage; tearing of the umbilical cord, placenta, or vasa previa; twin-twin transfusion; or rupture of an abdominal viscus.

Infants in shock usually demonstrate tachycardia of greater than 180 beats per minute (although bradycardia is not unknown), tachypnea, and signs of hypotension. The latter include pallor (although pinkness and cyanosis also may occur) and poor capillary filling (non-pinking up of "fingerprints" pressed into the skin). These infants look sick.

Immediate measures are stabilization of ventilation and treatment of asystole or bradycardia as described above. Any infant requiring treatment for shock should be transferred to a hospital for subsequent care. Rarely is such therapy appropriate in the home. The umbilical vein is catheterized and intravenous solutions given in an initial dose of 10 ml/kg as a rapid "push." Colloid solutions such as 5% albumin are preferred. However, any solution (including normal saline, half-strength lactated Ringer's, 5% dextrose in water) is acceptable during transport.

Asphyxia of the Newborn and Meconium Aspiration

The asphyxiated term fetus usually expels meconium into the amniotic fluid. Asphyxia also stimulates intrauterine respiratory movements, which can result in aspiration of amniotic fluid containing meconium into the oropharynx and upper respiratory tree. With the first few breaths after birth, this meconium can be sucked deeper into the lungs, with resultant chemical pneumonia.

The passage through ruptured amniotic membranes of thick meconium at any time during labor is an indication for transfer to a hospital. The passage of thin meconium in the latent phase of labor has different prognostic implications and does not signify increased risk for the newborn (see discussion in Chapter 11).

Whether in home or hospital, the passage of meconium is an indication for vigorous suctioning of the mouth, larynx, and nose with the DeLee suction catheter immediately after the birth of the head and prior to initiation of respiration. There is some controversy over the relative merits of the DeLee and the bulb syringe with respect to provoking cardiac arrhythmias in the newborn.[5] In practice, the DeLee, with its superior suctioning capability, has won wide acceptance despite this objection.

If meconium is recovered from the oropharynx (and even if it is not, according to some authorities) the standard recommendation is to visualize the larynx and to mouth-suction the trachea with either the DeLee or an endotracheal catheter. Catheterization and aspiration of the trachea are repeated until the returns are clear of meconium. Tracheal suction is a relatively safe procedure, while meconium aspiration can be a serious problem, warranting all efforts at prevention.

Even if the infant has already clearly aspirated meconium, suctioning the oropharynx and trachea until clear is recommended to minimize further aspiration. Following airway suction, the gastric contents should also be suctioned by passing the DeLee catheter via the nose through the esophagus to stomach. Otherwise, stomach contents can be regurgitated and aspirated.

THE NEWBORN EXAMINATION

The most critical initial observations to be made at a birth are those included in the Apgar scoring system detailed earlier in this chapter. These same observations are also included in the more comprehensive newborn examination that routinely occurs within an hour after the birth, when the third stage and perineal care are completed and the parents have had a chance to be with the baby. Only the highlights of this initial physical examination will be covered here. For more information the reader is referred to standard texts.

Color

Newborns should be pink, not blue, yellow, or white except for possible duskiness of the hands, feet, and (occasionally) lips. Color in dark-skinned newborns is best determined in the mucous membranes of the mouth.

Respiration

The breathing rate is normally between 40 and 60 per minute. In contrast to older children and adults, infants are periodic breathers. They may breathe regularly and then cease entirely for five to ten seconds, or the rate may vary. During normal periodic pauses the color remains stable. Changes in color with pauses define apneic spells, which are pathological.

Breathing should be easy, not labored. Retractions, flaring of the nostrils, and grunting are characteristics of labored (i.e., abnormal) breathing.

Listening to the lungs with a stethoscope in an infant with normal respirations and color is not particularly revealing. Significant respiratory disease in the absence of tachypnea is rare unless the central nervous system also is malfunctioning.

Neurological Examination

Much of the neurological assessment is done in the course of the general examination. Symmetry of movement, posture, and muscle tone are noted, as are response to handling (crying and quieting) and the qualities of the cry (normal or high or low pitched). During crying the facial muscles can be observed for evidence of weakness.

The grasp reflexes are tested by placing the examiner's index fingers in the baby's palms. With each hand the infant's fingers are then grasped between the examiner's index finger and thumb. The body is raised to a sitting position. The degree of head lag and control is noted, taking into account that a crying infant will often toss its head back. The baby is maintained in the sitting position momentarily and the trunk moved forward and backward enough to test head control once again. Even the newborn should exhibit some head control; the head should not bob like a ball on a stick. Next the head and trunk are allowed to fall back slowly to the mattress. Just before head contact, the examiner's fingers are released from the infant's hands and the infant is permitted to fall the rest of the way, activating the Moro reflex.

Cardiac Examination

The heart examination should be performed only when the infant is quiet. The chest is palpated to determine whether the heart is on the right or left side. The heart rate normally ranges between 120 and 160 beats per minute and varies according to the baby's state of arousal. Murmurs are very common in the newborn and usually represent normal shifts in circulation, such as the closing of the ductus arteriosus. On the other hand, even serious cardiac defects may not produce murmurs. In an asymptomatic infant, observation over time is the most useful determinant of the source of a murmur. The femoral pulses should be palpated with the baby quiet. They usually can be felt even though they can be quite weak.

Abdominal Examination

The abdominal examination of the newborn is facilitated by the normal laxity of the musculature and by the relative absence of air in the intestines. The baby should be quiet. An effective approach is to begin with gentle pressure on stroking from the lower to upper abdomen on each side to identify the edges of the liver, spleen, and other masses. The newborn's liver normally extends 2 to 2.5 cm below the rib margin. Deep palpation should follow. During the first several days the kidneys should be identifiable.

Genital Examination

The genitalia are inspected and palpated. The external genitalia should look normal. Ambiguity requires immediate consultation for clarification regarding sex assignment.

The male usually has a marked phimosis and a foreskin that fully covers the glans. Lesser or partial degrees of coverage by the foreskin, particularly when associated with location of the urethral meatus at a site other than the tip of the penis, should arouse concern. The examiner works the testes down into the scrotum from the internal ring on each side of the upper shaft of the penis. They should be of equal size. Hydroceles are common and usually disappear with time.

In the female the labia are normally swollen at birth. A creamy white vaginal discharge is common, as is a pseudomenses after the second day. The examiner spreads the labia to look for imperforate hymen, cysts of the vaginal wall, and masses within the labia.

Back, Extremity, and Joint Examination

Back, extremities, and joints are examined in turn. With the baby held face down in the hand, the length of the spine from nape of neck to coccyx is inspected for sinus tracks and soft midline swellings suggestive of meningoceles or other abnormalities. Since the shape of the bones of the baby at birth reflects intrauterine pressures, tibial bowing and passively correctable forefoot adduction are common. On the other hand, fixed (i.e., noncorrectable) positions of the forefoot or heel deserve immediate orthopedic evaluation.

The examiner checks for dislocation of the hip by placing the infant in a frog-leg position on its back on a flat surface with the examiner's third fingers on the acetabulae and thumbs and index fingers grasping the knees. A superiorly and posteriorly dislocated hip is demonstrated by palpably reducing it through pushing simultaneously upward with the third finger and downward and laterally with the thumb.

Head, Neck, and Mouth Examinations

Moulding of the head is common and in itself is of no clinical significance. Swelling of the skin and subcutaneous tissue of the head (caput succedaneum) is due to pressure during labor and characteristically bridges over a suture line. In contrast, swelling due to bleeding between skull and periosteum (cephalohematomas) is confined by the suture lines where the periosteum firmly attaches to bone. Mobility of the suture lines is tested by pushing with the thumbs on each side of the line. Immobility suggests craniostenosis. The neck is inspected for masses (usually midline), webbing, length, and mobility (to exclude torticollis). The mouth is checked for clefts in the gum and palate and for the presence of teeth. Small white inclusion cysts known as Epstein's pearls, usually in the midline near the juncture of the hard and soft palates, are normal. A tight frenum ("tongue-tie") may interfere with nursing.

Determination of Maturity

Determination of maturity is made by assessing the baby's physical and functional development according to established standards (Figure 12-1).

Eye Examination

Eye examination consists of inspecting the conjunctivae for hemorrhages, checking the cornea for lucidity (the cornea should always be

Figure 12-1 Newborn Maturity Rating and Classification

(A) ESTIMATION OF GESTATIONAL AGE BY MATURITY RATING
Symbols: X - 1st Exam   O - 2nd Exam

NEUROMUSCULAR MATURITY

	0	1	2	3	4	5
Posture						
Square Window (Wrist)	90°	60°	45°	30°	0°	
Arm Recoil	180°		100°-180°	90°-100°	< 90°	
Popliteal Angle	180°	160°	130°	110°	90°	< 90°
Scarf Sign						
Heel to Ear						

PHYSICAL MATURITY

	0	1	2	3	4	5
SKIN	gelatinous red, transparent	smooth pink, visible veins	superficial peeling &/or rash, few veins	cracking pale area, rare veins	parchment, deep cracking, no vessels	leathery, cracked, wrinkled
LANUGO	none	abundant	thinning	bald areas	mostly bald	
PLANTAR CREASES	no crease	faint red marks	anterior transverse crease only	creases ant. 2/3	creases cover entire sole	
BREAST	barely percept.	flat areola, no bud	stippled areola, 1-2 mm bud	raised areola, 3-4 mm bud	full areola, 5-10 mm bud	
EAR	pinna flat, stays folded	sl. curved pinna, soft with slow recoil	well-curv. pinna, soft but ready recoil	formed & firm with instant recoil	thick cartilage, ear stiff	
GENITALS Male	scrotum empty, no rugae		testes descending, few rugae	testes down, good rugae	testes pendulous, deep rugae	
GENITALS Female	prominent clitoris & labia minora		majora & minora equally prominent	majora large, minora small	clitoris & minora completely covered	

Gestation by Dates _____ wks

Birth Date _____ Hour _____ am / pm

APGAR _____ 1 min _____ 5 min

MATURITY RATING

Score	Wks
5	26
10	28
15	30
20	32
25	34
30	36
35	38
40	40
45	42
50	44

SCORING SECTION

	1st Exam=X	2nd Exam=O
Estimating Gest Age by Maturity Rating	_____ Weeks	_____ Weeks
Time of Exam	Date _____ am Hour _____ pm	Date _____ am Hour _____ pm
Age at Exam	_____ Hours	_____ Hours
Signature of Examiner	M.D.	M.D.

Figure 12-1 continued

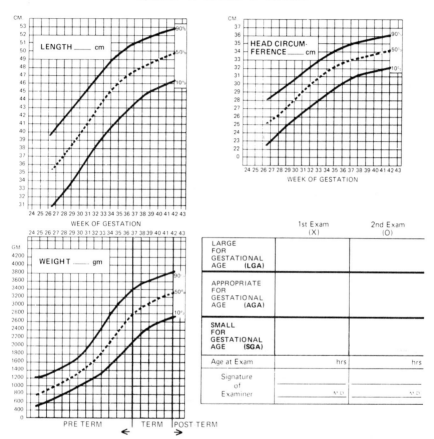

CLASSIFICATION OF NEWBORNS –
(B)   BASED ON MATURITY AND INTRAUTERINE GROWTH
Symbols: X · 1st Exam   O · 2nd Exam

	1st Exam (X)	2nd Exam (O)
LARGE FOR GESTATIONAL AGE **(LGA)**		
APPROPRIATE FOR GESTATIONAL AGE **(AGA)**		
SMALL FOR GESTATIONAL AGE **(SGA)**		
Age at Exam	hrs	hrs
Signature of Examiner	M.D.	M.D.

Sources: (a) Reprinted from "Classification of the Low-Birth-Weight Infant," by A.Y. Sweet, in *Care of the High-Risk Infant,* 2nd ed., Marshall H. Klaus and Avroy A. Fanaroff, with permission of W.B. Saunders Co., © 1977.

(b) Adapted from "Intrauterine Growth in Length and Head Circumference as Estimated from Live Births at Gestational Ages from 26 to 42 weeks," by L.O. Lubchenco, C. Hansman, and E. Boyd, *Pediatrics,* vol. 37, p. 403–408, with permission of the American Academy of Pediatrics, © 1966, and from "A Practical Classification of Newborn Infants by Weight and Gestational Age," by F.C. Battaglia and L.O. Lubchenco, *Journal of Pediatrics,* vol. 71, pp. 159–163, with permission of C.V. Mosby Co., © 1967.

clear, not cloudy), and identifying the red reflexes of the retina with an ophthalmoscope. Some examiners prefer to defer search for the red reflexes until the first examination following birth.

Head Circumference, Body Length, and Weight

Head circumference, body length, and weight are usually determined at the end of the examination. The full-term newborn's head circumference is between 33 and 37 cm (13 and 15 inches), and the length is 48 to 53 cm (19 to 21 inches). The baby can be weighed conveniently with a portable hook-type scale. The baby is wrapped in a tightly knotted receiving blanket suspended by the hook attached to the scale.

Summary of Conditions Requiring Prompt Early Attention

Findings on the examination, apart from those related to cardiorespiratory function, which warrant prompt early attention include the following:

- jaundice (see following section)
- major congenital anomalies such as omphalocele, meningomyelocele, hydrocephalus, and cyanotic congenital heart disease
- abdominal masses
- orthopedic abnormalities: clubfoot, metatarsus adductus, and dislocated hip
- absence of the red reflex in one or both eyes
- ambiguous genitalia
- seizures, apneic spells, choking, vomiting, hypotonia, fever, irritability, weak or high-pitched cry, and other signs of neonatal stress

The reader is referred to standard works on these subjects. All birth attendants should be aware of the problems of sepsis, pneumonia, meningitis, hypoglycemia, and hypocalcemia in the newborn.

JAUNDICE

The differential diagnosis of jaundice in the newborn is well covered in standard texts. Jaundice occurring within the first 24 hours of life signifies a rate of rise of bilirubin sufficiently high that intervention will be necessary. The infant so affected deserves a full evaluation and probably is a candidate for hospitalization. Standard nomograms[6] for the management of hyperbilirubinemia should be used in consultation with a neonatologist. Such guidelines should, however, be interpreted in the context of other indicators of the infant's well-being, since bilirubin level by itself is a very imprecise predicator of neonatal outcome.

Most parents are inexperienced in recognizing and assessing jaundice. Accordingly, it is advisable for the attendant to evaluate jaundice during postpartum home or office visits (see Chapter 13). Deep jaundice should be quantified with bilirubin measurements.

Home treatment of a jaundiced baby includes exposure to daylight, often recommended as a form of natural phototherapy for the baby with elevated bilirubin levels (usually estimated clinically). Although this approach seems logical, its effectiveness has not been firmly established.

There is also no evidence that extra water promotes excretion of bilirubin.

DEATH OF A NEWBORN

Despite the attendants' best efforts, the possibility of either a stillbirth or a postpartum death exists in any home or hospital birth. Few experiences can instill such a sense of sadness and helplessness in the attendants. Nevertheless, they must be prepared to help the family cope with tragedy.[7-9] In this regard the home setting can be used to advantage in that it obviates the need to deal with institutional procedures and unfamiliar hospital personnel, however sensitive these individuals might be to the needs of parents in such a crisis.

If a baby is clearly dead at birth (limp, cyanotic, absent heart beat, no respirations), this fact should be announced without any effort at resuscitation or transfer to hospital being made. If resuscitation of a depressed liveborn fails before transfer can be achieved, the resuscitation should stop, and the parents should be informed of the death. Physicians and midwives may have to approach such situations differently. Physicians have the legal authority to decide that death has occurred, while midwives in most areas are obliged to initiate and continue resuscitative efforts until medical attention is obtained.

The focus then shifts to coping with the death. Under these circumstances the guiding principles of care are to assist the parents in dealing with the reality, to encourage their full communication of feelings, beliefs, and fantasies, and to support them in fully grieving the loss.

The parents should be encouraged to look at and hold the baby, by themselves if they so wish. Photographs are useful for later recall. Naming the child can help concretize the baby's having been alive. Crying should be accepted fully, not denigrated. The attendants, too, can feel free to vent their feelings, including crying.

The medical examiner should be notified. If an autopsy is requested by the examiner, the attendants can support this request in that an autopsy will provide the parents with more information to explain the tragic outcome. The attendants should know under what conditions an autopsy is required by state law. They should also make clear that they will share the results of the postmortem examination with the parents.

Parents may be encouraged to plan a funeral and burial or cremation even if they would not be motivated to do so on religious or other grounds. The funeral serves to concretize the death and allows the parents to feel the support of friends and relatives. Funeral and burial services for infants generally are not expensive.

Many resources are available to help families cope with stillbirth or infant death, both immediately and in the months that follow. Books for families on this subject are listed in Appendix C. There is an organization called Aiding a Mother Experiencing Neonatal Death (AMEND) (see Appendix A), and additional resources are available from the International Childbirth Education Association (see Appendix B).

Some Implications of the Death of an Infant

The death of an infant, which is one of the worst outcomes of a birth from both the clinical and personal points of view, also has political overtones. Opponents of home birth are likely to use a death as evidence against the safety of home birth. It is both common and appropriate for family and attendants to question their own judgment. Inevitably the couple will ask themselves whether the tragic outcome could have been avoided had they been in a hospital. The possibility that the home setting has contributed to the death is one reason for having had the discussion of risk during the first or second prenatal meeting (see Chapter 7).

For the benefit of all parties concerned—the couple, the attendants, the medical profession, and governmental authorities—the authors' policy has been to encourage review of any mishap. We have found that an aboveboard approach, including maintenance of compiled statistics, has invariably served to increase our credibility and manifest our sense of responsibility, even to detractors. Ultimately the movement to reestablish home birth must rest on the truth. In that way all who evaluate home birth will have facts, not rumors, to work with. Furthermore, it is only through rigorous scrutiny of one's own actions that improvements in judgment and technique will occur.

NOTES

1. Marshall H. Klaus and John H. Kennell, *Maternal-Infant Bonding: The Impact of Early Separation or Loss on Family Development* (St. Louis: C.V. Mosby, 1976).

2. Virginia Apgar, "A Proposal for a New Method of Evaluation of the Newborn Infant," *Anesthesia and Analgesia* 32 (1953): 260–267.

3. Michael F. Epstein, Ivan D. Frantz III, and Gerald W. Ostheimer, "Resuscitation in the Delivery Room," in Joint Program in Neonatology (John P. Cloherty and Ann R. Stark, eds.), *Manual of Neonatal Care* (Boston: Little, Brown, 1980), pp. 55–69.

4. Paul B. Jennings, Errol R. Alden, and Ronald W. Brenz, "A Teaching Model for Pediatric Intubation Utilizing Ketamine-Sedated Kittens," *Pediatrics* 53 (1974): 283–284.

5. Herman A. Hein and Albert D. Warshauer, "Management of Neonatal Asphyxia," *Journal of the American Medical Association* 243 (1980): 2482–2483.

6. Marshall H. Klaus and Avroy A. Fanaroff, *Care of the High-Risk Neonate,* 2nd ed. (Philadelphia: W.B. Saunders, 1979), p. 259.

7. William T. Speck and John H. Kennell, "Management of Perinatal Death," *Pediatrics in Review* 2 (1980): 59–62.

8. William L. Hildebrand and Richard L. Schreiner, "Helping Parents Cope with Perinatal Death," *American Family Physician* 22, no. 5 (November 1980): 121–125.

9. Elizabeth Kirkley-Best and Kenneth R. Kellner, "Grief at Stillbirth: An Annotated Bibliography," *Birth and the Family Journal* 8, no. 2 (Summer 1981): 91–99.

Chapter 13

Postpartum Care

Principal Author: Peggy Spindel, R.N.

In the United States we should do more to improve the quality of support given after a baby is born. In England, the district midwife is required by law to visit a new mother every day for 10 days.[1] In Holland, home health aides are available to every home birth mother.[2-4] Yet in the United States, there is usually no postpartum contact after the hospital stay until the six-week checkup. In a home birth practice, continued contact is essential.

A midwife usually has more time than a physician for this close followup. Her experience as a woman and the quality of the relationship built up with the family over the preceding months add to the appropriateness of the midwife's primary role at this time. However, there are many ways in which different members of the home birth team can be useful to the family after the birth. A male physician can provide an example of a concerned and nurturing male figure that will support the father in his adjustment and encourage all family members to share in responsibility for the child. The physician-parent or midwife-parent is in a good position to support working parents.

Two basic elements of a successful postpartum followup are good preparation before birth and good communication afterwards. Childbirth classes and birth attendants should give parents information on what to expect and what to watch for. General recommendations for self-care are outlined at the end of this chapter. The birth attendant should be thoroughly familiar with the details of general nursing care after birth. Before the birth attendant leaves the home after the birth, she should be sure the family is settling in well and that breast-feeding has begun. She should summarize the parents' responsibilities, when she expects them to call her, and when she will return. We recommend home visits by the midwife on the first and third days and actively encourage frequent phone contact with the parents for at least a week. The parents also bring the baby to the office for the phenylketonuria heel prick (Guthrie test) on the fourth or fifth day.

(In somes states a test for hypothyroidism is included.) Sometimes a midwife will do this test in the home. Of course, any other schedule that provides good contact and that suits families and attendants is acceptable.

The goals of postpartum care revolve around the new mother, for when her needs are met, appropriate loving care to the newborn follows naturally. A mother who feels good about herself will communicate security to the baby and enhance a positive self-image in the developing child. Therefore, the mother needs good food, rest, and emotional support so that her body can return to its nonpregnant state and so that she can establish successful lactation. Dana Raphael has introduced the term *doula*[5] or mother supporter to suggest that a new mother herself needs a mother figure to support her, especially in the learned art of breast-feeding. A woman having a home birth has the unique opportunity to select a doula from her family, friends, caregivers, or resources like La Leche League, and to have this doula involved from the birth onward.

The best credentials a birth attendant can have to counsel breast-feeding mothers are her own personal breast-feeding experiences, a deep commitment to the value of unrestricted breast-feeding,[6] and knowledge of normal variations in breast-feeding, including the needs of the working mother who wishes to breast-feed. If the attendant lacks the personal experience, as in the case of a male physician, he should work with a woman who has breast-fed as well as learning from his clients and from the growing literature on breast-feeding. If a midwife or nurse is not available, La Leche League or the Nursing Mothers' Council of the International Childbirth Education Association (ICEA) should be relied on. Even an experienced midwife with children of her own should not hesitate to establish close ties with a good lay breast-feeding counselor or group. Health Education Associates provides continuing education in breast-feeding for nurses and many excellent educational materials for parents.

POSTPARTUM HOME VISITS

A postpartum home visit is a combined physical examination and social call. The postpartum period is a time to absorb the uniqueness of every family situation; it is when families and practitioners alike reap the full benefits of the experiences they have shared. Appreciation of the family's strengths and skills should be verbalized. First-time parents in particular need encouragement to see themselves as competent caregivers to their babies. Advice from attendants should be consistent, well timed, and sensitive to the emotional vulnerability of new parents. Notwithstanding the temptation to impose models of behavior that conform to the way the midwife raised her family or the way the physician was trained, it is imperative that the attendant allow each new mother and each family to find their own way. Aside from the necessary physical checks, simply sitting with the mother, admiring the baby with her, and answering questions are often the best ways to help her solve her difficulties and gain confidence.

Examination of Baby

The baby is examined briefly for color, respiration, signs of distress, eye discharge, jaundice, dehydration, and cephalohematoma or other birth injury. Parents are questioned about sleep, feeding, and the passage of urine and meconium. The adequacy and appropriateness of the baby's care is usually apparent. Breast-feeding is observed. No baths or any other direct care need be given by the birth attendant.

Jaundice

If the home birth attendant has any question about the severity of jaundice, serum bilirubin determinations should be performed and the baby assessed by a physician. The baby should be observed in strong daylight. The skin should be blanched by pressure to see true color. Obviously a deep orange or bronze is more severe than a lighter yellow. Jaundice usually is mild when it only covers the head and trunk, moderate when it also covers the arms and legs, and severe when it includes the palms and soles.[7] For moderate jaundice in a baby who is nursing well and seems well hydrated, we suggest home phototherapy. This involves either bright daylight or full-spectrum plant lights for 15 minutes every hour, exposing and rotating the baby's body and protecting the eyes. A physician should be consulted about jaundice in an infant under 24 hours of age, about jaundice with lethargy, dehydration, or other abnormal signs, and about jaundice persisting after seven days.

Breast-feeding

Breast-feeding is observed if at all possible. The attendant should look for proper positioning of the baby (belly to belly with the mother) and comfortable maternal posture. The mother may welcome suggestions for nursing while lying down so that she can doze. The attendant should look for proper nursing technique, that is, proper positioning of the nipple in the baby's mouth and proper tongue and gum action on the part of the baby. The presence of engorgement, leaking milk, the "let-down" reflex, gulping sounds made by the baby while nursing, and frequent wet diapers (six or more per day) all indicate that the milk has "come in" and breast-feeding is established. The attendant must be able to recognize normal patterns of nursing and the variety of normal "nursing personalities" of babies.[8,9]

The attendant should be alert for problems in breast-feeding such as the following:

- infrequent nursing (intervals greater than three hours, total nursings fewer than eight per day). The attendant should be prepared to make suggestions for getting the baby to breast-feed more often.
- too frequent nursing. Nursing once or twice per hour around the clock may, in some women, ultimately lead to reduced milk supply. Although this can be a normal pattern of nursing, the attendant can still make suggestions for keeping the baby at breast longer and lengthening the intervals between feedings.
- sore and cracked nipples
- breast infections

In the unlikely event that the mother chooses not to breast-feed, even for a few days, she should select an appropriate formula with the help of the attendant. Binding the breasts or at least firm support will make her more comfortable as she awaits the drying up of the milk. In addition, the woman's uterine involution should be watched more closely. Bromocriptine (Parlodel®) and danocrine (Danazol®) have also been used to stop lactation.

Examination of Mother

The mother should be asked about her general well-being, rest, nutrition, ease of urination, and amount and character of lochia. Her fundus is palpated and her vulva and breasts briefly examined. Blood pressure and temperature are taken as needed. In the authors' experience, we have never needed to catheterize a new mother or had a postpartum infection. These problems should be very rare in a home birth practice. Secondary postpartum hemorrhage and vascular complications are also rare. The reader is referred to standard obstetrics and midwifery texts for treatment of these problems.[10,11] Urinary tract infections and hemorrhoids are treated as in pregnancy but usually with more success.

Excessive blood loss at the delivery should be monitored by hematocrits and responded to through nutritional counsel. The mother should be reminded that foods high in protein, vitamin C, and calcium are important, in addition to iron for red cell production. If the hematocrit is low at four to five days, iron supplementation may be considered.

General Observations

The birth attendant should be on the alert for the occasional distressful problems of the postpartum period. Various combinations of physical and psychological problems can precipitate a family crisis in the days and weeks following birth. A sluggish baby who will not nurse and a mother who is exhausted and painfully engorged, with sore nipples, is one such combination. A screaming baby, intervening and undermining grandparents, and parents who feel frazzled and incompetent is another. The "superwoman" with older children who refuses to stop waiting on everyone else long enough to care for herself is a candidate for problems. Such situations, which can become nightmarish, call for a more active approach on the part of the birth attendant. Daily visits are helpful: to assess the family's needs, to provide loving support, and to offer concrete suggestions. The mother should be encouraged to get into bed and take the baby with her. Relatives, friends, or prenatal class members can be mobilized to bring cooked food, do laundry and shopping, and care for other children while the parents focus on their problem. For those who are obsessively neat, the view that people should have priority over things can be suggested. If the family is beseiged by well-wishers, brief visiting hours can be arranged and the phone taken off the hook. In some communities paid postpartum home help is available. A referral to a postpartum support group (where available) is wise. Even after initial problems are solved, new parents can still be at risk and need to know they are not alone.

Several types of postpartum support may be available. One is an independent counseling group such as C.O.P.E. (Coping with the Overall Pregnancy Experience) in the Boston area. Often childbirth preparation organizations, such as the local affiliates of ICEA, or home birth classes have reunions or continuing workshops. If need be, a home birth practice can organize its own programs, ranging from an informal group discussion to a structured class series. The main feature should be to provide a forum for new parents to meet others with whom they can share their feelings and concerns and can support and educate each other.

POSTPARTUM OFFICE VISITS

Traditionally the postpartum checkup is done six weeks after the birth, although for breast-feeding mothers four weeks is also an option, because involution is usually quick. The mother often comes with her baby, and if another family member is not present, some provision should be made for the baby's care during the pelvic examination.

A hematocrit and urine culture are obtained, as well as weight and blood pressure. (For a woman who has lost a lot of blood, a hematocrit would also have been done at the time of the phenylketonuria test.) Inquiries are made about bleeding, breast-feeding, family adjustments, and sexual activity. A breast examination is done and a once-a-month self-examination is encouraged, even though the woman is breast-feeding. A full pelvic examination is done to rule out subinvolution or gynecological problems such as cystocele or rectocele and to assess the healing of the perineum and the return of the tone of the pelvic floor. (The examiner should be aware that the speculum may be the first thing that the woman has had in her vagina since the birth.) The examiner will commonly note a mild atrophy (thinness, smoothness, tenderness) in the vaginal mucosa of breast-feeding women. If this normal, self-limiting condition is observed, the woman and her partner should be reminded that the discomfort during intercourse that may result can be alleviated by using a water-soluble lubricant such as K-Y jelly. This is also a good time to stress the need for further practice of the Kegel exercises and to evaluate the condition of the abdominal muscles. If a disposable plastic speculum is used, it can be offered to the woman for subsequent self-examination.

The attendant discusses birth control and the return of fertility, being sure to note that ovulation can occur before a menstrual period. Although the contraceptive effect of breast-feeding may be taken into account in family planning, breast-feeding is not in itself as reliable as other contraceptive methods (except when practiced with an extreme frequency rarely seen in this country). A diaphragm can be fitted during this six-weeks' postpartum office visit, although it may need to be refitted several months later. Other methods may require a separate appointment. Natural family planning is an option, although it is usually taught after the return of menstruation.

The postpartum checkup is also an appropriate time to look back on the birth, to evaluate how it was handled by both family and caregivers, and to assess the implications for future pregnancies. If a complication occurred that puts the woman into a high-risk category, planning for other options can begin immediately. If a problem arose that is unlikely to be repeated, such as breech presentation, the parents need to feel confident that they can look forward to a normal birth next time. In any case, these issues should become a part of an ongoing dialogue between parents and caregivers.

Although not every woman is ready or willing to share deeply private thoughts and feelings, the birth attendant should indicate that she is interested in what the woman, her partner, and other family members perceive as the meaning of the birth process for them. Women and their families are to be encouraged to write down their memories. Thoroughly digesting the birth experience can help them move on to the next phase of their lives. Sometimes serious disappointments come to light that take a long time to resolve.

The home birth attendant may find herself an integral part of the meaning of birth for a woman. Although such participation is probably the deepest pleasure a birth attendant can feel—to be part of the love and joy and pain and pride of birth—the birth is something the woman herself has accomplished, and the attendant must clearly acknowledge her for it.

POSTPARTUM SELF-CARE FOR FAMILIES

Postpartum care is, for the most part, self-care. The following outline lists areas in which families should be instructed in postpartum maternal and infant care. It is based on a postpartum guide written by parents in the childbirth education group Birth Day (see Chapter 8) in collaboration with the midwives and physicians in the authors' practice. Information on the subjects listed may be obtained from the organizations and recommended readings for families included in the Appendices.

Immediate Care after Birth

- proper maternal bowel and bladder habits
- checking uterine fundus and monitoring bleeding
- hygiene and perineal care
- perineal pain relief
- diet (including fluid intake)
- Kegel exercises
- jaundice in the newborn
- bathing the newborn
- cord care
- normal urine and meconium in the newborn
- clothing the newborn
- eye care for the newborn
- nipple care and breast-feeding
- nursing relationship between mother and babý

Postpartum Issues

- incorporating the birth experience
- feelings of parental inadequacy
- postpartum blues and "mothering the mother"
- mental and emotional changes
- sibling relationships and rivalry
- sexual interest, physical changes affecting sexual functioning, and family planning

---

NOTES

1. Margaret F. Myles, *Textbook for Midwives,* 8th ed. (Edinburgh: Churchill Livingstone, 1975), pp. 624–625.

2. Suzanne Arms, *Immaculate Deception; A New Look at Women and Childbirth in America* (Boston: Houghton Mifflin, 1975), p. 271.

3. Neal Devitt, "Hospital Birth Versus Home Birth: The Scientific Facts, Past and Present," in David Stewart and Lee Stewart (eds.), *Compulsory Hospitalization: Freedom of Choice in Childbirth?* (Marble Hill, Mo.: NAPSAC, 1979), pp. 499–500.

4. W.G. Van Arkel, A.J. Ament, and N. Bell, "The Politics of Home Delivery in the Netherlands," *Birth and the Family Journal* 7 (1980): 101–112.

5. Dana Raphael, *The Tender Gift: Breastfeeding* (New York: Schocken Books, 1976), pp. 24, 147–161.

6. Ruth A. Lawrence, *Breastfeeding: A Guide for the Medical Profession* (St. Louis: C.V. Mosby, 1980), p. 7.

7. Lewis Barness, *Manual of Pediatric Physical Diagnosis* (Chicago: Year Book Medical Publishers, 1972), pp. 185–186.

8. Raphael, *The Tender Gift.*

9. Lawrence, *Breastfeeding.*

10. Jack A. Pritchard and Paul C. MacDonald, *Williams Obstetrics,* 15th ed. (New York: Appleton-Century-Crofts, 1976), pp. 374–384, 757–783.

11. Myles, *Textbook for Midwives,* pp. 396–413.

Professional and Support Organizations

Aiding a Mother Experiencing Neonatal Death (AMEND)
c/o Mrs. Maureen Connelly, Coordinator
4325 Berrywick Terrace
St. Louis, Missouri 63128

Alternative Birth Crisis Coalition
P.O. Box 48371
Chicago, Illinois 60648

American Academy of Husband-Coached Childbirth (AAHCC)
Box 5224
Sherman Oaks, California 91413

American College of Home Obstetrics
P.O. Box 25
River Forest, Illinois 60305

American College of Nurse-Midwives
1522 K Street, N.W., Suite 1120
Washington, D.C. 20005

American Foundation for Maternal and Child Health
30 Beekman Place
New York, New York 10022

American Physical Therapy Association
1111 North Fairfax Street
Alexandria, Virginia 22314

ASPO/LAMAZE
1840 Wilson Blvd., #204
Arlington, Virginia 22201

Association for Childbirth at Home International (ACHI)
P.O. Box 39498
Los Angeles, California 90039

Boston Women's Health Book Collective
P.O. Box 192
West Somerville, Massachusetts 02144

C/SEC
(Cesareans/Support, Education and Concern)
22 Forest Road
Framingham, Massachusetts 01701

Cooperative Birth Center Network (CBCN)
Box 1, Rt. 1
Perkiomenville, Pennsylvania 18074

Coping with the Overall Pregnancy Experience (COPE)
37 Clarendon Street
Boston, Massachusetts 02116

Couple to Couple League
P.O. Box 11084
Cincinnati, Ohio 45211

Frontier Nursing Service
Wendover, Kentucky 41775

Home-Oriented Maternity Experience (HOME)
P.O. Box 450
Germantown, Maryland 20874

Informed Homebirth, Inc.
P.O. Box 788
Boulder, Colorado 80306

International Childbirth Education Association (ICEA)
P.O. Box 20048
Minneapolis, Minnesota 55420

International Planned Parenthood Federation
Western Hemisphere Region
105 Madison Avenue
New York, New York 10016

La Leche League International Inc.
9616 Minneapolis Avenue
Franklin Park, Illinois 60131

Maternity Center Association
48 East 92nd Street
New York, New York 10028

NAPSAC International
(InterNational Association of Parents and Professionals for Safe
Alternatives in Childbirth)
P.O. Box 267
Marble Hill, Missouri 63764
(NAPSAC maintains an extensive list of home birth support
organizations throughout the world.)

Nursing Mothers' Council
Boston Association for Childbirth Education
726 Washington Street
Whitman, Massachusetts 02382

Physicians for Automotive Safety
P.O. Box 208
Rye, New York 10580

Materials Obtainable by Mail

For *Bookmarks,* a catalog of recommended readings prepared by the ICEA, write:
ICEA Bookcenter
P.O. Box 20048
Minneapolis, Minnesota 55420

A similar catalog of readings entitled *Imprints* is available from:
Birth and Life Bookstore
7001 Alonzo Avenue N.W.
P.O. Box 70625
Seattle, Washington 98107

For the booklet entitled "Children at Birth" by Jenifer M. Fleming, send $3 and self-addressed manila envelope to:
Birth Day
P.O. Box 388
Cambridge, Massachusetts 02138

For the booklet "Midwifery and the Law" by Pacia Sallomi, Angie Pallow-Fleury, and Peggy O'Mara McMahon (from *Mothering*), send $3.50 to:
Mothering Publications, Inc.
P.O. Box 2208
Albuquerque, New Mexico 87103-2208

For information about the Midwives' Alliance of North America, contact:
    Concord Midwifery Service
    30 South Main Street
    Concord, New Hampshire 03301

"Higgins Intervention Method for Nutrition Rehabilitation During Pregnancy" is available from:
    Montreal Diet Dispensary
    2182 Lincoln Avenue
    Montreal, Quebec H3H 1J3
    Canada

The booklet *As You Eat So Your Baby Grows* by Nikki Goldbeck is available for $1.50 (sample copy free to health professionals) from:
    Ceres Press
    Box 87, Department P
    Woodstock, New York 12498
Bulk and professional discounts are available upon request.

The booklet *Nutritional Guidelines for Pregnancy and Lactation* is available from:
    California Department of Health Services
    714–744 P Street
    Sacramento, California 95814

Information about prenatal breast preparation is available from:
    Health Education Associates
    211 South Easton Road
    Glenside, Pennsylvania 19038

Information about giving up smoking is available from:
    Office of Cancer Communications
    National Institutes of Health
    Room 10718
    Bethesda, Maryland 20205

Instructional visual aids on the physiology of pregnancy and fetal development are available from:
    Maternity Center Association
    48 East 92nd Street
    New York, New York 10028

Instructional visual aids on the physiology of labor and birth are available from:
Midwest ParentCraft Center
627 Beaver Road
Glenview, Illinois 60025

Instructional visual aids on all phases of childbirth education for parents and professionals are available from:
Childbirth Graphics
P.O. Box 17025
Irondequoit Station
Rochester, New York 14617

Audiovisual aids and books on pregnancy, childbirth, and parenting are available from:
Educational Graphic Aids
1315 Norwood
Boulder, Colorado 80302

Birth attendants' equipment and parents' supplies are available from:
Cascade Birthing Supply
P.O. Box 76
Marion, Oregon 97359

Electronic perineometers are available from:
Health Technology Inc.
50 Lawn Avenue
Portland, Maine 04103

For a free copy of "The Pregnant Patient's Bill of Rights," send a self-addressed stamped envelope to:
Committee on Patient's Rights
Box 1900
New York, New York 10001

"Don't Risk Your Child's Life" is available for 50¢ from:
Physicians for Automotive Safety
P.O. Box 208
Rye, New York 10580

Appendix C

Suggested Readings

BOOKS FOR PROFESSIONALS

Obstetrics Textbooks

Cavanagh, Denis; Woods, Ralph E.; and O'Connor, Timothy C.F. *Obstetric Emergencies*. 2nd ed. Hagerstown, Md.: Harper & Row, 1978.

Friedman, Emanuel A. *Labor: Clinical Evaluation and Management*. 2nd ed. New York: Appleton-Century-Crofts, 1978.

Garrey, Matthew M.; Govan, A.D.T.; Hodge, Colin; and Collander, R. *Obstetrics Illustrated*. 3rd ed. New York: Churchill Livingstone, 1980.

Llewellyn-Jones, Derek. *Fundamentals of Obstetrics and Gynaecology. Volume I: Obstetrics*. 2nd ed. London: Faber and Faber, 1977.

Niswander, Kenneth. *Obstetrics: Essentials of Clinical Practice*. 2nd ed. Boston: Little, Brown, 1981.

Oxorn, Harry. *Oxorn-Foote Human Labor and Birth*. 4th ed. New York: Appleton-Century-Crofts, 1980.

Pritchard, Jack A., and MacDonald, Paul C. *Williams Obstetrics*. 16th ed. New York: Appleton-Century-Crofts, 1980.

Reeder, Sharon R.; Mastroianni, Luigi, Jr.; Martin, Leonide L.; and Fitzpatrick, Elise. *Maternity Nursing,* 14th ed. New York: Harper & Row, 1980.

Romney, Seymour L.; Gray, Mary Jane; Little, A. Brian; Merrill, James A.; Quilligan, E.J.; and Stander, Richard. *Gynecology and Obstetrics: The Health Care of Women*. 2nd ed. New York: McGraw-Hill, 1981.

Midwifery Textbooks

Davis, Elizabeth. *A Guide to Midwifery: Hearts and Hands*. Santa Fe: John Muir Publications, 1981.

Gaskin, Ina May. *Spiritual Midwifery.* Rev. ed. Summertown, Tenn.: The Book Publishing Co., 1978.

Myles, Margaret. *Textbook for Midwives.* 9th ed. New York: Churchill Livingstone, 1981.

Varney, Helen. *Nurse-Midwifery.* Boston: Blackwell Scientific Publications, 1980.

General Historical and Methodological Works

*Bursztajn, Harold; Feinbloom, Richard I.; Hamm, Robert M.; and Brodsky, Archie. *Medical Choices, Medical Chances: How Patients, Families, and Physicians Can Cope With Uncertainty.* New York: Seymour Lawrence/Delacorte, 1981.

Ehrenreich, Barbara, and English, Deirdre. *Witches, Midwives and Nurses: A History of Woman Healers.* Oyster Bay, N.Y.: Glass Mountain Press, 1973.

*Wertz, Richard, and Wertz, Dorothy C. *Lying-in: A History of Childbirth in America.* New York: The Free Press, 1977.

Pregnancy and Childbirth

Burrow, Gerard N., and Ferris, Thomas F. *Medical Complications During Pregnancy.* Philadelphia: W.B. Saunders, 1975.

Kitzinger, Sheila. *Education and Counseling for Childbirth.* New York: Schocken Books, 1979.

Kitzinger, Sheila, and Davis, John A., eds. *The Place of Birth.* New York: Oxford University Press, 1978.

Peterson, Gayle H. *Birthing Normally: A Personal Growth Approach to Childbirth.* Berkeley, Calif.: Mindbody Press, 1981.

Shanteau, Doreen, ed. *Audiovisuals About Birth and Family Life, 1970–1980.* Minneapolis: International Childbirth Education Association, 1981.

Shrock, Pamela; Ellis, Judith; Bunnin, Nenelle; and Shearer, Madeleine, eds. *Directory of Instructional Materials in Childbirth and New Parent Education.* 2nd ed. Berkeley, Calif.: Birth, 1982.

Watt, Bernice K., and Merrill, Annabel L. *Handbook of the Nutritional Contents of Foods.* New York: Dover Publications, 1975.

---

*May also be of interest to families.

Postnatal and Pediatric Care

Barness, Lewis. *Manual of Pediatric Physical Diagnosis*. 5th ed. Chicago: Year Book Medical Publishers, 1980.

Cloherty, John P., and Stark, Ann B., eds. *Manual of Neonatal Care*. Boston: Little, Brown, 1980.

*Klaus, Marshall H., and Kennell, John H. *Parent-Infant Bonding*. 2nd ed. St. Louis: C.V. Mosby, 1981.

Lawrence, Ruth. *Breastfeeding: A Guide for the Medical Profession*. St. Louis: C.V. Mosby, 1980.

BOOKS FOR FAMILIES

Prenatal Nutrition, Exercise, and Well-Being

Brewer, Gail S., and Brewer, Tom. *What Every Woman Should Know: The Truth About Diet and Drugs in Pregnancy*. New York: Random House, 1977; New York: Penguin, 1979.

Clark, Linda. *Know Your Nutrition*. Rev. ed. New Canaan, Conn.: Keats Publishing, 1981.

Dilfer, Carol. *Your Baby, Your Body*. New York: Crown, 1977.

Goldbeck, Nikki. *As You Eat So Your Baby Grows*. Woodstock, N.Y.: Ceres Press, 1977.

Noble, Elizabeth. *Essential Exercises for the Childbearing Year,* 2nd ed. rev. Boston: Houghton Mifflin, 1982.

Parvati, Jeannine, and O'Brien, Medvin. *Prenatal Yoga and Natural Birth*. Felton, Calif.: Freestone, 1978.

Robertson, Laurel; Flinders, Carol; and Godfrey, Bronwen. *Laurel's Kitchen: A Handbook for Vegetarian Cookery and Nutrition*. Petaluma, Calif.: Nilgiri Press, 1976; New York: Bantam Books, 1978.

Shandler, Nina, and Shandler, Michael. *Yoga for Pregnancy and Birth: A Guide for Expectant Parents*. New York: Schocken Books, 1979.

Simkin, Diana. *The Complete Pregnancy Exercise Book*. New York: New American Library, 1980.

Williams, Phyllis C. *Nourishing Your Unborn Child*. New York: Avon, 1975.

Pregnancy and Childbirth

Arms, Suzanne. *Immaculate Deception: A New Look at Childbirth in America*. Boston: Houghton Mifflin, 1975; New York: Bantam, 1977.

Baldwin, Rahima. *Special Delivery*. Millbrae, Calif.: Les Femmes Publishing, 1979.

Bean, Constance. *Labor and Delivery: An Observer's Diary*. New York: Doubleday, 1977.

Bean, Constance. *Methods of Childbirth: A Complete Guide to Childbirth and Maternity Care*. 2nd rev. ed. New York: Doubleday, 1982.

Bing, Elisabeth. *Six Practical Lessons for Easier Childbirth*. Rev. ed. New York: Bantam, 1977.

Bing, Elisabeth, and Colman, Libby. *Making Love During Pregnancy*. New York: Bantam Books, 1977.

Bittman, Sam, and Zalk, Sue Rosenberg. *Expectant Fathers*. New York: Ballantine, 1980.

Boston Association for Childbirth Education. *Handbook in Prepared Childbirth*. Rev. ed. Wayne, N.J.: Avery Publishing Group, 1981.

Boston Women's Health Book Collective. *Our Bodies, Ourselves: A Book by and for Women*. Revised and expanded. New York: Simon and Schuster, 1983.

Bradley, Robert A. *Husband Coached Childbirth*. New York: Harper & Row, 1965.

Brewer, Gail S. *The Pregnancy after 30 Workbook*. Emmaus, Pa.: Rodale Press, 1978.

Dick-Read, Grantly. *Childbirth Without Fear*. Rev. 4th ed. New York: Harper & Row, 1978.

Ewy, Donna, and Ewy, Rodger, *Guide to Family-Centered Childbirth*. New York: Dutton, 1982.

Haire, Doris. *The Cultural Warping of Childbirth: A Special Report*. Minneapolis: International Childbirth Education Association, 1972.

Hazell, Lester. *Commonsense Childbirth*. Rev. ed. New York: Tower Publications, 1976.

Home-Oriented Maternity Experience. *A Comprehensive Guide to Home Birth*. Washington, D.C.: Home-Oriented Maternity Experience, 1976.

Hotchner, Tracy. *Pregnancy and Childbirth: The Complete Guide for a New Life*. New York: Avon Books, 1979.

Kitzinger, Sheila. *Birth at Home*. New York: Oxford University Press, 1979.

Kitzinger, Sheila. *The Complete Book of Pregnancy and Childbirth*. New York: Alfred A. Knopf, 1980.

Kitzinger, Sheila. *The Experience of Childbirth*. New York: Penguin, 1978.

Kitzinger, Sheila. *Giving Birth: The Parents' Emotions in Childbirth.* New York: Schocken Books, 1970.

Lang, Raven. *The Birth Book.* Palo Alto, Calif.: Genesis Press, 1972.

Leboyer, Frederick. *Birth Without Violence.* New York: Alfred A. Knopf, 1975.

Leboyer, Frederick. *Loving Hands.* New York: Alfred A. Knopf, 1976.

Milinaire, Caterine. *Birth: Facts and Legends.* New York: Harmony Books, 1974.

Milunsky, Aubrey. *Know Your Genes.* Boston: Houghton Mifflin, 1977.

Nilsson, Lennart. *A Child Is Born.* Rev. ed. New York: Delacorte, 1977.

Noble, Elizabeth. *Childbirth with Insight.* Boston: Houghton Mifflin, 1983.

Noble, Elizabeth. *Having Twins: A Parent's Guide to Pregnancy, Birth and Early Childhood.* Boston: Houghton Mifflin, 1980.

Parfitt, Rebecca Rave. *The Birth Primer.* New York: New American Library, 1980.

Petty, Roy. *Home Birth.* Northbrook, Ill.: Quality Books, 1979.

Simkin, Penny. *Directory of Alternative Birth Services and Consumer Guide.* 2nd ed. Marble Hill, Mo.: NAPSAC, 1980.

Simkin, Penny, ed. *Kaleidoscope of Childbearing: Preparation, Birth and Nurturing.* Seattle: the pennypress, 1978.

Sousa, Marion. *Childbirth at Home.* New York: Bantam Books, 1977.

Stewart, David, and Stewart, Lee. *Compulsory Hospitalization: Freedom of Choice in Childbirth?* 3 vols. Marble Hill, Mo.: NAPSAC, 1979.

Stewart, David, and Stewart, Lee. *The Five Standards for Safe Childbearing.* Marble Hill, Mo.: NAPSAC, 1981.

Stewart, David, and Stewart, Lee. *Safe Alternatives in Childbirth.* 3rd ed. Marble Hill, Mo.: NAPSAC, 1978.

Stewart, David, and Stewart, Lee. *21st Century Obstetrics Now!* 2 vols. Marble Hill, Mo.: NAPSAC, 1977.

Tanzer, Deborah, and Block, Jean L. *Why Natural Childbirth? A Psychologist's Report on the Benefits to Mothers, Fathers and Babies.* New York: Schocken Books, 1976.

Ward, Charlotte, and Ward, Fred. *The Home Birth Book.* Washington, D.C.: Inscape Publishers, 1976.

White, Gregory. *Emergency Childbirth.* Philadelphia: Police Training Foundation, 1958.

Young, Diony. *Changing Childbirth: Family Birth in the Hospital.* Rochester, N.Y.: Childbirth Graphics Ltd., 1982.

Cesarean Birth

Cohen, Nancy Wainer, and Estner, Lois J. *Silent Knife: Cesarean Prevention and Vaginal Birth after Cesarean*. South Hadley, Mass.: J.F. Bergin, 1983.

Donovan, Bonnie. *The Cesarean Birth Experience*. Boston: Beacon Press, 1978.

Hausknecht, Richard, and Heilman, Joan R. *Having a Cesarean Baby*. New York: E.P. Dutton, 1978.

Young, Diony, and Mahan, Charles. *Unnecessary Cesareans: Ways to Avoid Them*. Minneapolis: International Childbirth Education Association, 1980.

Breastfeeding

Brewster, Dorothy Patricia. *You Can Breastfeed Your Baby . . . Even in Special Situations*. Emmaus, Pa.: Rodale Press, 1979.

Eiger, Marvin, and Olds, Sally. *The Complete Book of Breastfeeding*. New York: Bantam Books, 1973.

Kippley, Sheila. *Breast-Feeding and Natural Child Spacing: The Ecology of Natural Mothering*. Rev. ed. New York: Harper & Row, 1974; New York: Penguin, 1975.

Kitzinger, Sheila. *The Experience of Breastfeeding*. New York: Penguin, 1980.

LaLeche League. *The Womanly Art of Breastfeeding*. 3rd ed. Franklin Park, Ill., 1981.

Montagu, Ashley. *Touching: The Human Significance of the Skin*. New York: Columbia University Press, 1971.

Nursing Mothers' Council of the Boston Association for Childbirth Education. *Breastfeeding Your Baby*. Rev. ed. Wayne, N.J.: Avery Publishing Group, 1981.

Pryor, Karen. *Nursing Your Baby*. Rev. ed. New York: Harper & Row, 1973.

Raphael, Dana. *The Tender Gift: Breastfeeding*. New York: Schocken Books, 1976.

Postpartum, Postnatal, and Pediatric Care and Parenthood

Boston Children's Medical Center and Feinbloom, Richard I. *Child Health Encyclopedia*. New York: Seymour Lawrence/Delacorte, 1978.

Boston Women's Health Book Collective. *Ourselves and Our Children: A Book by and for Parents*. New York: Random House, 1978.

Brazelton, T. Berry. *Infants and Mothers: Individual Differences in Development*. New York: Delacorte, 1969; New York: Dell, 1972.

Brazelton, T. Berry. *Toddlers and Parents: A Declaration of Independence*. New York: Delacorte, 1974.

Brewer, Gail S., and Greene, Janice. *Right from the Start: Meeting the Challenges of Mothering Your Unborn and Newborn Baby*. Emmaus, Pa.: Rodale Press, 1981.

Colman, Arthur, and Colman, Libby. *Earth Father, Sky Father: The Changing Concept of Fathering*. Englewood Cliffs, N.J.: Prentice-Hall, 1981.

DelliQuadri, Lyn, and Breckenridge, Kati. *Mother Care*. New York: Pocket Books, 1979.

Fraiberg, Selma. *The Magic Years*. New York: Scribner's, 1968.

Friedland, Ronnie, and Kort, Carol, eds. *The Mothers' Book: Shared Experiences*. Boston: Houghton Mifflin, 1981.

Hale, Nathan Cabot. *Birth of a Family: The New Role of the Father in Childbirth*. Garden City, N.Y.: Doubleday, 1979.

Howell, Mary. *Healing at Home: A Guide to Health Care for Children*. Boston: Beacon Press, 1979.

Howell, Mary. *Helping Ourselves: Families and the Human Network*. Boston: Beacon Press, 1975.

Kitzinger, Sheila. *Women as Mothers: How They See Themselves in Different Cultures*. New York: Random House, 1980.

Newton, Niles. *The Family Book of Child Care*. New York: Harper & Row, 1957.

Nofziger, Margaret. *A Cooperative Method of Natural Birth Control*. Rev. ed. Summertown, Tenn.: The Book Publishing Co., 1978.

Pantell, Robert H.; Fries, James F.; and Vickery, Donald M. *Taking Care of Your Child: A Parent's Guide to Medical Care*. Reading, Mass.: Addison-Wesley, 1977.

Pizer, Hank, and Garfink, Christine. *The Post Partum Book: How to Cope With and Enjoy the First Year of Parenting*. New York: Grove Press, 1979.

Rozdilsky, Mary Lou, and Banet, Barbara. *What Now? A Handbook for New Parents*. New York: Charles Scribners and Sons, 1975.

Samuels, Mike, and Samuels, Nancy. *The Well Baby Book*. New York: Summit Books, 1979.

Thevenin, Tine. *The Family Bed: An Age Old Concept in Childrearing.* Minneapolis: Thevenin, 1976.

Loss and Grieving

Berezin, Nancy. *After a Loss in Pregnancy.* New York: Simon and Schuster, 1982.

Borg, Susan O., and Lasker, Judith. *When Pregnancy Fails: Families Coping with Miscarriage, Stillbirth, and Infant Death.* Boston: Beacon Press, 1981.

Friedman, Rochelle, and Gradstein, Bonnie. *Surviving Pregnancy Loss.* Boston: Little, Brown, 1982.

Schiff, Harriet S. *The Bereaved Parent.* New York: Penguin, 1978.

Schweibert, Pat, and Kirk, Paul. *When Hello Means Goodbye.* Portland, Ore.: University of Oregon Health Sciences Center, 1981.

PERIODICALS

American Journal of Obstetrics and Gynecology
Birth (formerly *Birth and the Family Journal*)
The Female Patient
International Journal of Obstetrics and Gynecology
Journal of Nurse-Midwifery
Journal of Perinatal Medicine
Journal of Reproductive Medicine
Mothering
NAPSAC News
Obstetrics and Gynecology
The Practicing Midwife
Women and Health

Index

I

About the Authors

STANLEY E. SAGOV, M.D., who received his medical degree at the University of Cape Town, South Africa, is a family physician in practice at Family Health Care in Cambridge, Massachusetts. He is on the faculty of the University of Massachusetts and Harvard Medical Schools and was formerly Associate Director of the Harvard Family Health Care Program. Dr. Sagov is the author of *The Active Patient's Guide to Better Medical Care* (1976) as well as textbook chapters and journal articles. He serves as a medical consultant to the Boston Association for Childbirth Education.

RICHARD I. FEINBLOOM, M.D., is Clinical Associate Professor of Family Medicine at the State University of New York at Stony Brook. A graduate of the University of Pennsylvania Medical School, he formerly directed the Family Health Care Program at Harvard Medical School and practiced family medicine in Cambridge, Massachusetts. He is the author, with the Boston Children's Medical Center, of *Child Health Encyclopedia* (1978) and a co-author of *Medical Choices, Medical Chances* (1981). Dr. Feinbloom is past president of Physicians for Social Responsibility and has been a consultant to the International Childbirth Education Association.

PEGGY SPINDEL, R.N., a practicing midwife since 1977, is the chairperson of the Massachusetts Midwives' Alliance. In 1975 she helped design childbirth education classes for Birth Day. She earned an Associate Degree in Nursing in 1978. A graduate of Brandeis University, she lives in Newton, Massachusetts, with her husband and three children.

ARCHIE BRODSKY is a professional writer specializing in medicine, psychology, and human services. He is co-author of *Love and Addiction* (1975), *Burnout: Stages of Disillusionment in the Helping Professions* (1980), *Medical Choices, Medical Chances* (1981), and *Sexual Dilemmas for the Helping Professional* (1982).

About the Contributors

GEORGE J. ANNAS, J.D., M.P.H., is the Edward Utley Professor of Health Law at Boston University School of Medicine and Chief of the Health Law Section of Boston University's School of Public Health. From 1976 to 1981 he served as vice-chairman of the Massachusetts Board of Registration in Medicine. He has authored a number of books on health law, including *The Rights of Hospital Patients* (1975) and *The Rights of Doctors, Nurses and Allied Health Professionals* (1981).

JENIFER M. FLEMING, B.A., Cert. Ed., has taught childbirth classes for Birth Day in the Boston area for several years. Having worked with families as a social worker and a preschool teacher, she came to childbirth education through her own experiences of birth. A native of Scotland, she has four daughters, all born with the help of midwives, the last two at home in Cambridge, Massachusetts.

JUDITH DICKSON LUCE has been active in the women's health movement for the past 10 years and has practiced for the past 6 years as a lay midwife, both independently and in conjunction with the authors of this book. She became involved with women's health care through her own childbirth experiences, particularly the home birth of her third child. She has contributed to symposia on childbirth sponsored by the National Science Foundation and by the National Association of Parents and Professionals for Safe Alternatives in Childbirth. She was a member of the Boston Task Force on Regionalization of Maternity Care.

ELIZABETH NOBLE, R.P.T., is Director of the Maternal and Child Health Center in Cambridge, Massachusetts. The founder and past chairwoman of the Obstetrics and Gynecology Section of the American Physical Therapy Association, she is the author of *Essential Exercises for the Childbearing Year* (2nd edition revised, 1982), *Having Twins* (1980), and *Childbirth with Insight* (1983).